ROLLERCOASTER

**How a man can survive
his partner's breast cancer**

Woody Weingarten

VitalityPress

ROLLERCOASTER

a must-read

This book is written with humor, humanity and great insight. It's way over-do and a must-read for all those who love someone experiencing the traumas of breast cancer.

— **RoyAnne Florence, Sonoma, California**

Thankfully our guide in this sadly familiar odyssey is an accomplished journalist. The reader is coaxed, buoyed, confounded, frightened, charmed and ultimately imbued with a sense of direction. Glance at any page at random and you will stumble on a helpful thought, a gem, even a tonic for the perplexed male caregiver.

— **Marc Machbitz, Honolulu, Hawaii**

Like a lot of men, my attitude toward life challenges has always been to address things head on and find a "fix." When my mother-in-law had aggressive cancer, my first stop was WebMD and Wikipedia, but ultimately neither of these gave any sort of real context or understanding of what my role could be. This book gives well-needed context and support for men dealing with these "unfixable" life challenges for the first time.

— **Robert Huebner, Melbourne, Australia**

Woody Weingarten's book is a love story that can benefit thousands of other men. It is about conquering the travails of a loved one's fight against a dread disease. It is a story of life, not just for the cancer survivor but for the forgotten person in the struggle, the partner of the survivor.

— **Gary Price, San Rafael, California**

Fantastic, sad, funny. Absolutely a joy to read.

— **Frances French, Armonk, New York**

ROLLERCOASTER

Woody Weingarten is right. My wife's journey, our journey, after her breast cancer diagnosis has been like a rollercoaster — fear, uncertainty and disorientation. But our ride has been made immeasurably easier by him having placed himself — with his book in his own voice — in the seat right next to us. His teachings show us we can overcome our fears, retain our hopes, and know our path has been illuminated by those who have faced similar challenges before us. His book is like a warm hand, reaching out to us, to our hearts, letting us know that we are not alone in our battle. Thank you, Woody, for your courage, strength and care, for telling us your story with the compassion and experience of a teacher, friend and survivor.

— **Stan Cohn, Kentfield, California;**
member, Marin Man to Man support group

Weaving between the battle his wife fought against breast cancer and their deeply romantic relationship as her treatment evolved, Weingarten paints a profound and fascinating story. The couple's effort is meaningful to us all, and provides the reader with real ways through the challenges. The author's writing is bold, his message intense and educational. Although the thrust of "Rollercoaster" is unusual in that the focus is on the partner rather than the patient, it should be of immeasurable benefit to both partners in a relationship.

— **Ivan Silverberg, M.D., oncologist,**
Laguna Honda Hospital, San Francisco, California

I've finished reading "Rollercoaster" and was impressed, moved and inspired. The book would be a gift for any male caregiver whose partner is dealing with breast cancer or any life-threatening disease. The author's relationship with his wife and the manner in which they dealt with her cancer are extraordinary, as is his ability to chronicle the experience. That's quite a parlay, and I think the result is a love story that has a great deal to say, not only to male caregivers but to anyone, male or female, who is a partner in a significant, intimate relationship.

— **Neil Levy, Sacramento, California**

ROLLERCOASTER

This book is a must-read for anyone affected directly or indirectly by breast cancer.

The author not only immerses the reader in the devastating impact of this all too common affliction and its treatment on his wife, but also in the emotional rollercoaster of his experience and of the other male partners of cancer patients in his men's group, a not often presented narrative. His superb writing skills lead us along the path of initial discovery, diagnosis, therapeutic and reconstructive surgery, chemotherapy and irradiation to emotional and physical rehabilitation. He also supplies a thoughtful, well-documented and informative discussion of the various treatment options and the supports available to patients, partners and loved ones. As a physician involved for 40 years in both the medical and emotional aspects of cancer treatment, I give "Rollercoaster" my most enthusiastic recommendation.

— **Kenneth G. Lerner, M.D., psychiatrist,**
Veterans Administration Medical Center, Manchester, New Hampshire;
staff physician, British Columbia Cancer Agency, Vancouver, B.C.

Published by VitalityPress
San Anselmo, California

No information in "Rollercoaster" is intended to be a diagnostic or treatment tool for any condition — or a substitute for advice or medical care from your personal physician. No reference constitutes or implies an endorsement of any kind. Readers should also be aware that websites or telephone numbers listed in this book might change without notice.

Rollercoaster and VitalityPress logos are trademarks of VitalityPress.

Print and ebook design by David Kudler, StillpointDigitalPress.com

Cover design: Edward Marson, edward@u-nique.me
Front cover photo: Larry Rosenberg, lrphoto.com
Back cover photo: Alan Babbitt, abproductions.com

Publisher's Cataloging-in-Publication
(Provided by Quality Books, Inc.)

Weingarten, Woody.
Rollercoaster : how a man can survive his partner's
breast cancer / Woody Weingarten. -- First edition.
152 pages 23 cm
Includes bibliographical references.
LCCN 2014954302
Print ISBN 978-0-9905543-0-1
Ebook ISBN 978-0-9905543-1-8

1. Weingarten, Woody. 2. Male caregivers--United
States--Biography. 3. Fox, Nancy, 1939- 4. Breast--
Cancer--Patients--United States--Biography. 5. Breast--
Cancer--Popular works. 6. Cancer--Patients--Family
relationships--United States.   I. Title.

RC280.B8W45 2014   616.99'44900922
                            QBI14-600180

10 9 8 7 6 5 4 3 2 1

VitalityPress

VitalityPress.com

CONTENTS

ROLLERCOASTER

1
FOREWORD

Blind to her power, the freckle-faced visitor from Detroit ignited my teenage hormones and escalated my awkwardness. I let the olive oil from the pizza dribble down my knuckles.

That made her giggle. The sound rolled across our table in the suburban New York City restaurant.

Red-haired Nancy Falk, a blink past 16 that winter, could accurately be labeled shy. I exhibited that trait, too, despite her envisioning me — a college freshman two years older — as a pinnacle of sophistication.

Her distorted view led me to a clichéd conclusion: We were meant for each other.

Sometimes I flash back to the misbelief that I, a six-footer who occasionally tripped over his size-13 sneakers, loved her instantly. But the truth is, I thought corresponding with her would help keep me sane at an upstate college during icy nights.

The next semester, however, I invited her to fly to a fraternity party at my school, Colgate University.

"Wow, a weekend with a real college man," she gushed to a girlfriend.

The party came and went uneventfully, both of us too skittish to do anything carnal. We had fun anyway, walking and talking and peeling off the outer philosophical layer of life, box-stepping across the dance floor, squirming to keep our noses from bumping when we kissed.

Perhaps it was her hazel eyes that snared me. Or the trendy flip of her hair. Whatever the allure, I was smitten.

And by the time the jet back to the Motor City swallowed her, we both knew. "This is eternal," I melodramatically proclaimed as she left.

"Eternal," she echoed.

Month after month stretched by. Letter writing eclipsed my studies and exams. Each night we'd both fall asleep, 374 air miles apart, imagining the next party weekend. When it finally arrived, I nervously attached my frat pin to her dress.

"*My God,*" thought Nancy the Innocent. "*Now I'll have to give him sexual liberties. He'll probably want to touch my bare breast.*"

Bulls-eye!

Several of my body parts throbbed with desire for even more. But I could wait: After all, we were engaged to be engaged.

My eyes scanned left and right; strange, no 20-piece orchestra appeared to play "My Funny Valentine," *our* song. But what the heck, we were pinned, and that alone guaranteed we'd be together forever, right?

Forever lasted until summer, when Nance found me sporting dark sunglasses, dark sandals and a white-hot desire to write. The package simply didn't match the wish list of a tallish girl from the Midwest with a slightly crooked smile. "Maybe you should marry a doctor instead of me," I suggested in reaction to her reaction.

Without guile or recognition of the triteness of the dialogue, she replied, "Maybe we *should* see some other people."

So we did. And lost touch. Completely.

Though the odds against such a coincidence seemed astronomical, she married a guy from my hometown high school class, a wannabe obstetrician-gynecologist. I wed a girl from a neighboring town who had a straighter smile and decidedly bigger breasts.

I fathered one kid of each gender; Nance gave birth to a daughter. Both of us hopscotched the country.

Fast-forward about three decades. Change the scene to Mill Valley, a small Northern California community. Tall redwood trees. Narrow, winding streets. Upscale houses with deer scampering across unfenced back yards. Red Porsches and black Beemers and white Mercedes. Quaint boutiques and coffee shops. Chic filmmakers and ex-hippies flaunting neck crystals. Several hills and one traffic jam north of San Francisco and the Golden Gate Bridge.

Tucked into a faceless shopping center was a homey pizzeria — uh huh, another pepperoni palace, the only kind of eatery the fates and I apparently patronize at moments of sublime impact.

I strolled to the bar for a Diet Pepsi. There stood Nance, 2,440 miles from Colgate, 2,079 miles from Detroit, a million miles from our youth, asking for the identical drink. Her face was wrinkled but her eyes illuminated a direct path to her identity. "Nancy Falk," I shouted, grinning idiotically. "Nancy Falk."

"Woody," she shouted back, "is that you in middle-aged makeup?"

We embraced. We chatted briefly — and, of course, awkwardly. "*Who the hell is this person?*" I wondered. "*Why has she time-warped back into my life?*"

She guided me to a table where her daughter was bonding with a pizza. The girl was almost the same age her mom had been when we met, but I saw no resemblance. Indeed, I could hardly see the teen at all; I was too busy staring at Nance's long, un-flipped red hair and laugh lines.

We lunched the next day, and gabbed on the phone a few times the following week. We covered through oral shorthand the events (including our respective divorces) that had matured us yet left us basically the same. After noting she was now Nancy Fox, having appropriated a grandmother's last name and discarded her ex's, she invited me home to share dinner.

The cartoonist she'd been living with for five years would be there, she said.

I entered the Twilight and Chutzpah Zones simultaneously. In the living room, as I clinked my Amaretto glass to hers, I handed Nance a gift, a small crystal pyramid I'd blithely inscribed on its base "Timeless love, Woody." She politely mumbled "Thanks" and positioned it on a coffee table.

All through the meal my gaze never left her high cheekbones. Her lover ceased to exist; my current bed partner never came to mind. When the evening ended, I still couldn't fathom why she'd returned to unravel my life.

"See ya soon," I muttered without conviction.

Before I could begin to solve what I labeled "the Nancy puzzle," my father's prostate cancer leapt from remission to metastases. Cancer. "*Is there a more terrifying word in the English language?*"

Life-threatening cells invaded every lymph node in his body and many of his bones. The prognosis: Death in the short run. So I returned to my childhood home in New Rochelle to help my mother cope, and to share his final days. I told only a handful of close friends where I was going; Nance wasn't among them.

Shortly after he died, peacefully and under his own roof five months later, I moved back to the San Francisco Bay Area and broke up with my sheetmate. Before long, weary of the seesaw economics of freelance writing and editing, I accepted a job managing a Jewish-community newspaper. It was a comfortable fit since I was starved for spiritual morsels as well as the company of others.

Nance subscribed to the weekly but infrequently read it. However, mindlessly sorting mail while on the phone one afternoon, she thumbed through the latest issue. An article about a rabbi advocating animal rights grabbed her attention. She noticed my byline.

Seconds later, she pressed the buttons of her touch-tone. "Where'd you disappear to?" she asked. I told her about the trip east. In a voice as fragile as one of the lace antimacassars that had protected my grandmother's furniture, she said, "Oh, I'm sorry. I'd thought you just didn't like me as a grown-up."

"No, no, of course I did," I said. "I do — like you, that is."

"Why don't we break bread together sometime," she suggested, her old-fashioned phrasing flustered me almost as much as the invitation.

"Sh-sh-sure. Okay."

I asked about her live-in. "He's moving out," Nance said.

Lunches followed, then dinners. We graduated to movies, and experienced the tiny weather variations San Franciscans call the passing of seasons. Friendship dates meant goodnight pecks on the cheek. No physical intimacy, no overnighters.

"This is ridiculous," I whined one day. "We're not kids anymore; we may even be on the cusp of old-farthood."

She promised to think about it.

Late one night a few weeks later we were nestled in a parked car swapping critiques of a screwball comedy we'd just seen. In what I've since learned is her standard-issue non sequitur style, Nance interjected, "Why are we here?"

"Holy Sartre, where'd that existentialism come from?" I thought. But I managed to quash my intellectual pomposity and ask instead, "Whadda ya mean, 'Why are we here?'"

"I mean, 'Why are we here rather than in your bed?'"

My studio apartment was 13 minutes away. I drove there in eight.

We enjoyed the coupling, but for countless new moons wrestled for control of the relationship. Both of us employed manipulative tricks honed as spoiled only-children. We played to a stalemate.

Volatility became our standard. One minute we'd acknowledge the depths of our love; an instant later, the friction would become palpable. Then, before anyone could say Sleeping Beauty and Prince Charming, we'd become a loving twosome again. So no one who knew us expressed surprise that, amid thousands crowding a holistic healing-metaphysical expo one sunny afternoon, I, the ultimate romantic, dropped without warning to one knee.

"Will you marry me?"

Nance almost joined me on the floor, her legs momentarily buckling. "We'll see," she said.

"Why do we always have to reverse roles?" I asked. "Men are supposed to be the ones who can't make a commitment."

"We'll see."

"But we were intended to be together," I continued, selling as fast and hard as I could. "We're soulmates. Why else would we have found each other again? There are 250 million people in the United States. You really think running into each other after all those years, all the way across the country, was a *coincidence?*"

Draw up a list of my character flaws and impatience will float to the top. I despise waiting. For anything. Especially anything important. So Nance's resistance pissed me off.

A year and a bit later, we bought a house and tested living together.

Shortly after my 50th birthday, we exchanged vows on our front deck.

A handful of friends watched our dog lap wine from the wedding chalice as the sun reflected off Nance's hand-painted silk gown. Her knees buckled again.

Several years went by faster than either of us could imagine, packed with all the usual whites, blacks and grays of life. "Change" and "challenge" became our personal buzzwords. We laughed a lot, and worked and worked at not messing up what Destiny had unquestionably blueprinted. "Missing years," I told a buddy, "have to be bridged, and ghosts of lovers-past erased."

A dual history had to be assembled one day at a time. Romance had to be nurtured.

We became so joyful working at being joyful that we never saw it coming. Just as we were getting the hang of living happily ever after, the diagnosis was every bit as unsettling as the big Loma Prieta earthquake had been:

Nance had breast cancer.

2

RELIEF

Nancy survived.

So did I, although I may have felt as delicate as an eggshell back then.

A full 20 years after Nance's diagnosis, we now focus day-to-day on the hundreds of mundane pleasures that fill the life of a post-cancer patient. We probably cram into our calendars a few too many social, cultural and civic activities. But every a.m. we make sure to say to each other, "Good morning — I love you."

And we love basking in the light at the end of the proverbial tunnel.

What a relief it is.

On the 10th anniversary of the final day of Nance's surgical, chemo-therapy and radiation endurance race, we clinked glasses of Diet Pepsi and drank to each other's good health.

Ditto, the 15th.

The 20th? Why fix what wasn't broken?

Our toasts were inspirational milestones, two, three or four times happier than the five-year benchmark oncologists and researchers delineate as the medical goal.

Now, since the odds of Nance dying in another 20 years or so from something *other than* breast cancer have increased exponentially, we've given ourselves permission to stop holding our collective breath. We savor our *joie de vivre*, a palpable difference from the times we bolted from anxiety to stress and back again. And we know a positive attitude can cause an immediate reversal of discontent.

I particularly remember the chilly December day I discovered a flat on the driver's side rear.

I cursed and called AAA.

A short time later, a lumber-hauler slid off the narrow road to our home and blocked the tow truck. I seethed, certain I'd be late to work.

After the disabled vehicle was pulled from the ditch and my nail-spiked tire changed, I drove to the San Francisco lot where I usually parked. A power company van was having trouble making a 180-degree turn. It blocked my car.

I swore again.

Yet it took only minutes — until I paid the attendant, a middle-aged woman who'd told me several weeks earlier she'd been stricken with ovarian cancer — to change my grumpy outlook with two brief sentences.

"Merry Christmas," she volunteered. "I'm happy to be alive."

Since then, I've learned to use the disease itself to brighten my demeanor.

Case in point: When someone dented my car while it was parked, I employed my new mantra, "Hey, it's not cancer."

From time to time my wife and I roll our eyes at the notion of 5-, 10-, 15- or even 20-year markers. Why would the day after any of those points be less risky for breast cancer patients than the previous 24 hours?

But rather than let our skepticism rattle us, we concentrate on the upbeat — including the idea of Nance earning a survivor badge each day by being mindful about what she eats, exercising consistently and checking in with physicians regarding unusual pains.

Proactive measures rank high for me as well, such as leading a support group for breast cancer partners where I can help show attendees how to hack through the underbrush of the breast cancer jungle.

Our website — Marin-Man-to-Man.org — explains why we meet weekly: The "emphasis is on making newcomers, and each other, feel less isolated, uncertain, misunderstood or afraid...[We look for ways] each man can reassure his partner that both she and their relationship are likely to survive...Through the good times and bad, most men loathe the stepchild-status breast cancer gives them. But the marvelous synergy of our group often acts as an antidote to that particular toxin."

That said, though, each participant must slay identical dragons: fear of his mate's quality of life dwindling or, worse yet, of her dying. One guy admits finding hope online when he "realized that Nancy was still alive...I stopped planning [my wife's] funeral."

At the same time, both Nance and I know that what we experienced two decades ago — both bad and good — is parallel to what most couples in similar circumstances face today.

And we may not have been able to predict it but we grew profoundly closer through her struggle with cancer and its aftermath.

That, in fact, is a typical outcome, though a small amount of couples — roughly one in ten — don't do so well and the tension breaks them apart.

Almost 250,000 U.S. women are diagnosed with breast cancer annually.

Which translates into roughly one every two minutes.

Americans, despite those daunting figures, don't have anywhere near the worst stats. Breast cancer strikes 39.4 per 100,000 in Iceland, almost double the incidence in the United States.

Still, more than 2 million stateside women live with the chronic disease and about 40,000 die of it each year (370,000 succumb worldwide).

According to the American Cancer Society, 13 percent of U.S. women (one in every eight) will get it at one point or another, and three-quarters of them will have no risk factors except that they're female.

A small percentage of males do get the disease, but that's a book for someone else to tackle.

It is important to note, however, that breast cancer tends to ignore the skin color, creed and sexual orientation of its targets.

And all things considered, it's crucial for hundreds of thousands of forgotten, invisible male caregivers to know they're not alone.

Given men's proclivity for thinking they require zero help and can fix anything, it's probable most would never even read about breast cancer without a nudge. But women — who typically have more than one male in their lives — instinctively realize their husbands, boyfriends, sons, fathers and brothers need support. So they push.

Nance gently nagged me to "try, just try" the men's group, accurately forecasting I'd become a regular if I found an outlet for my insecurities, doubts and pain.

To visualize what I went through as a caregiver, it's necessary, first, to recognize the malady as an enemy invisible to the naked eye, usually painless in the early stages. But then picture us in a bumpy rollercoaster climbing from the lows of the illness to the heights of the Great Wall of China.

These pages will show how a pair of very-human beings overcame their anguish in the wake of relentless medical procedures. It's not an abbreviated "10 Helpful Hints" on coping, but, instead, it integrates a running "how-to" account that can help distraught and proactive men (and their partners) pull back the translucent curtains of diagnosis, treatment and recovery.

Our journey certainly will illustrate that physical and psychological hurdles can be cleared, that strong relationships can help kill not only mutated cells but also the worries that metastasize, and that wellness can spring from research, healing and support networks.

It's a trip that's a partial memoir-chronicle, partial love story and cumulative guide to hope.

While this book is aimed at men, it also can give a woman some insight into what her male caregiver is experiencing. It could also be of value to anyone helping a loved one battle *any* life-threatening disease.

A while ago, a nearby hospital's cancer-care coordinator set up a focus group for me, mainly to see if we could learn why Marin Man to Man drop-ins had decreased in recent years. Her contention was all support-group attendance was falling because of readily available information on the Internet, despite much of it being inaccurate.

What happened surprised neither of us.

Several men who'd promised to come didn't show up, and those who did echoed a single theme: I don't need no stinkin' support group. I can deal with it alone.

One mid-lifer epitomized that posture. He didn't look anyone in the eye the entire session, and failed to raise his head while spewing all-too-common lies: "I have no questions. I don't treat my wife any differently. We're very happy."

Each fellow danced around denial by offering rationales for being uninterested in *any* group.

"At first I was really scared but now I've settled into a routine," said one.

"Very few of my friends know — my wife didn't want to tell and I don't either," explained another.

"I want to keep this positive and just move on," emphasized a third. "I need to spend more time with my kids, who treat it like any other disease, like head lice."

Although none hung up his machismo cape, one guy did sideswipe vulnerability by admitting he didn't "really know what my needs are."

A Canadian report confirmed not long ago that partners of breast cancer patients want to keep their lives as normal as possible and tend to look elsewhere for balance — to hanging out with friends or exercise, for example, rather than reaching out to support groups for help.

The experiences of Man to Man members belie that attitude, but we all readily admit it's a personal choice.

In contrast to the Canadian study and the focus group opinions, I clearly remember my own compulsion to crawl through the inferno. So

I have no trouble being open these days. Ditto for Nance, who recently commented, "I'm still vulnerable — *all the time.*"

We both may eagerly confront reality now, but I do recollect stuffing a ton of feelings during our first encounters with breast cancer hell.

And even today I periodically re-experience the sensation that the anguish stemming from a loved one's ailments can be so much worse than that triggered by one's own infirmity.

I recall, too, walking in molasses for weeks after Nance's diagnosis before I could absorb any real degree of relevant information. (What I indeed needed, and got soon enough, was what I dubbed a "Cancer College crash course" that led not to genuine knowledge at first but to a faux patina of expertise.)

My initial numbness had to taper off before I could be there for Nance no matter what, before I could inject humor into our bleakest moments, and before I could say "yes, dear" copiously and mean it.

Only then could I concoct my short but meaningful list for others:

- Patients sometimes prefer we listen in silence and squeeze their hand. Do just that.
- Get out of the way so help can pour in from friends, co-workers and health pros (females in particular).
- Learn what it is our partners truly want (the truth usually can be obtained simply by asking).
- Gather data or act as an *auxiliary* questioner, advocate and note-taker (polar opposites of the customary male role as chief problem-solver).
- Develop psychological skills to prick any thought-balloons that contain the notion our circumstances or emotions are unique. (My reactions and attitudes, and Nance's, actually mirrored those of ever so many patients and the 37 million caregivers who minister to the health needs of companions, kinfolk, friends or neighbors.)
- Pay attention to our own health and needs (every bit as imperative as the desire to care for our women).
- Figure out how to ward off verbal attacks from our partners stemming from their myriad fears and the sensation that they've lost control of their lives. They may, in any given moment, simultaneously consider us their best friends and worst enemies, though they most likely won't admit the latter.
- Plan something positive for a treatment-free future, something we'll both look forward to, whether it's a big-deal foreign trip or a little-deal date for a neighborhood movie.
- Eliminate negativity and avoid naysayers.

How I got there may be foggy but I can't forget letting go of my anger at doctors for not having instant answers, at pharmaceutical companies for manufacturing life-extending but not necessarily life-saving drugs, at myself for not having a magic wand.

While immersed in the struggles, we weren't convinced Nance would survive 20 months much less 20 years.

Fear more than half filled my glass.

I was petrified breast cancer would be my wife's killer. Yet she's flourishing today, as am I.

She even avoided what, according to a 2013 article in The New York Times, 70 percent of cancer survivors experience: "depression at some point."

And she didn't even need to consult with one of the survivorship-care programs that are popping up all over the country.

When her dermatologist spied an early-stage melanoma on Nance's left arm some time ago, we hired a surgeon to cut it out immediately. Another specialist, not long afterwards, identified two malignancies on my prostate. Hormone shots, radiation and a minor surgical procedure followed.

"We've lived through two of your cancers," I said to Nance. "Now we get to live through one of mine. "

Poet Robert Frost once declared that, in three words, he could "sum up everything I've learned about life: It goes on!"

Given the pinpoint vision of hindsight, that viewpoint is easy. But when a life-threatening crisis is gnawing at you, such pithy wisdom may be as hard to seize as a feather in a windstorm.

Panic, I remember, was the best I could muster when Nance's breast cancer was diagnosed.

3
SURGERY

There's no way my wife or I could have foreseen how tightly we'd be strapped into the cancer rollercoaster, the best metaphor for the unwanted trip we'd take together. But the journal excerpts in this chapter reflect just how unsteady, how jagged, the ride was.

Friday, Nov. 18

I slouched in the tiny waiting room of the surgical floor. Stomach knotted. Hands quivering. Mind in meltdown. His words bounced off the walls of my brain; I refused to let them take hold. "Nancy's all right but the tumor was cancerous."

His second sentence — "We believe we got it all" — couldn't undo the first.

"What does that mean?" "Will she be okay?" "For how long?" The questions rattled in my head.

"She's still asleep," the surgeon continued. "She doesn't know yet."

"Oh, God. Why her? Why her?"

I couldn't cry. I couldn't scream. I desperately wanted to do both.

The odds, the doctor had told us going in, were five chances in six the tumor would not be malignant. Nance beat the numbers, negatively. *"Will I ever trust statistics again?"*

The medical man in scrubs who'd just slipped me the bad news as unemotionally as if he'd been a weather guy reporting an overcast day left for another surgery. Twenty minutes evaporated as I mindlessly thumbed a handheld poker game. A nurse materialized and said I could see my wife.

She lay in a Marin General Hospital bed in Greenbrae, California, with a tube up her nose and an intravenous needle in her arm.

I stood there, hunched over, rehearsing what I'd say when she awakened.

Terror gnawed at my stomach. I didn't want to tell her. The doctor ought to do it. He'd undoubtedly had plenty of practice.

My anger at him intensified, even if he were purely the messenger, even if he'd preserved her life. Anyone who crossed my path now was potential prey. And if I couldn't find a human being to blame, I'd fault an invisible, monstrous, unkind God.

The surgeon reappeared shortly after Nance came out of the anesthetic. In a voice as flat as Kansas, he told her the findings of her lumpectomy.

Her eyes dulled. She said nothing for a few seconds but then crackled questions faster than he could reply. He eventually deflected the barrage by saying the painkiller would impair her memory. And he sidestepped her fear of needing her breast removed in spite of the surgery she'd just had. "It would be better if we discussed all this in my office in a few days," he said.

The man of medicine did answer a few minor queries — two or three times each because Nance forgot by the end of the series what she'd been told at the beginning. The process amused me, unquestionably a defense mechanism to ward off my anxiety. I broke into my first smile since the nightmare began.

The doc indicated we could expect at least one more operation — the removal of lymph nodes. "We'll talk about the rest later," he said.

The total impact of that phrase, "the rest," didn't register at first.

Saturday, Nov. 19

Sleeplessness plagued me all last night. My mind circled and circled, like a race driver pushing a car to the limit on a fast and dangerous track. My body writhed from one side of our king-size bed to the other.

At irregular intervals, when Nancy would visit her mom in Detroit or fly elsewhere on a business trip, I'd slept alone without difficulty. Now it felt different. The bed had become too spacious, too empty. The noise of one horrific thought overlapping another deafened me (*"until death do us part"*).

I strained to imagine what she was going through. I couldn't.

My thoughts became unreal. Though my apprehension was being replicated like paper in a copier gone haywire, it seemed secondhand, remote; hers surely must be magnified, right in her face.

I hoped Nance would be cured, and that 25 or 30 years from now she'd still be cancer-free. But this morning her right breast exhibited a bruise of many hues, largely purple with brown and yellow accents. It had marginally swollen.

"It's enormous," she said.

I was tickled by her temporarily having one puffy tit and one regular, but would I be so tolerant if it were my testicles instead? No way, José!

When she first undraped the boob for me, I stiffened. The gash extended a few inches. I inspected it with my eyes, afraid to touch it lest a microbe on my fingertips infect the wound. After staring for a few seconds, I relaxed.

"BFD, big fucking deal," I said, hoping to lessen her tension. "If that's the worst that'll happen, we're lucky as hell."

She grinned.

Sunday, Nov. 20

Nancy's right breast itched last night to a point of alarm.

She awoke in our bedroom at 2:30 a.m. convinced she was having a severe allergic reaction to the tape on her wound. She kvetched and kvetched, and finally agreed to call the surgeon. He, cursedly, had snuck away for the weekend.

Nance, wanting to be considerate to the on-call doctor, had suffered mutely until 7. The physician, unaware of that thoughtfulness, responded, according to my spouse, "in an extremely nasty manner — that she wasn't dressed and couldn't get to the hospital immediately."

Nance growled "fergeddit," and slammed the phone into its cradle. After all, aren't healers supposed to be a Hippocratic 911 available at the drop of a stitch?

"How 'bout driving to Marin General's emergency room?" I asked.

"No," replied my fifty-something wife. She wanted no medical novices treating a complication they might not yet have encountered.

We re-read the printed instructions the surgeon's staff had given us. The outer dressing could come off two days after the procedure; a series of strips over the incision should stay on; a hot shower would be okay. We checked our calendars, clocks and minds. "Go for it," I said.

Nance gently peeled back tape and gauze, overcoming a snowballing urge "to tear it off."

The shower rivaled Nirvana, sprinkling her with the lofty adult pleasure that comes from waiting an eternity for a good thing. As she scrubbed away the tape gum, the itching began to subside.

When it totally disappeared, our mutual anger about the cancer needed a new target. The on-call doc fit perfectly.

We spent a full five minutes using her as an oral dartboard.

Monday, Nov. 21

I buried myself in my job, editing at the Jewish Bulletin of Northern

California, hoping the routine hustle-bustle there might curb my jumpiness. (Holy shit! Writing the word "buried" really upset me just now. My fingers trembled on the keyboard. *Why can't I focus on life instead of death?"*)

While I registered over-the-top on the nervousness scale, Nance was mostly steeped in denial. She read voraciously but dozed often, overcome "by everybody talking about survival rates" — and, by implication, non-survival rates.

Examinations ate up her waking hours today: bone scan, chest X-ray, blood tests for liver and lungs. She drove to the site alone, after her surgeon pooh-poohed the risk of her incision opening should she have to brake suddenly. Nance also picked up her medical records from her gynecologist, to hand off to the cancer team.

"I was amazed at all the problems I've had with medications," my wife commented. "It made me anxious about cancer therapy."

Tuesday, Nov. 22

Sex crept back into our lives last night. Nancy initiated.

Despite her valiant attempt to bring a semblance of normalcy to our lives, despite my orgasm, it didn't satisfy. "This one-sidedness makes me squirmy, a little uncomfortable," I said.

"Me, too," Nance agreed.

The whole truth? Both of us were preoccupied.

Today, she and I apprehensively visited the surgeon to learn the test results. Instantaneous relief: He said her "margins were clear." That meant the pathologists had found no cancer cells within the perimeter of the removed tumor. The conclusions confirmed his speculation that he "got it all." Nance wouldn't lose her breast. No mastectomy.

The relief lasted only seconds, though, as he outlined the assorted side effects of the chemotherapy and radiation that were probable down the road.

Nance and I became mush-brains on the spot. Our ability to reason just oozed out and we substituted a comfort zone where we'd do whatever the gentle, cherub-faced, white-haired cutter suggested.

When we thought about it later, we couldn't quite pinpoint when we'd converted him from mortal to godhead — or ourselves into automatons. We did identify, however, that we'd consciously redefined my role: I was charged with locating a magic wand to repair any life patterns that might break down because of the cancer.

At the same time, I had to negotiate a mine-field of spats Nance put in our way, intentional diversions from her non-verbalized, internalized trepidation.

Whenever she could suck me into a squabble, she'd relish the opportunity to chastise me in ultra-proper 19th century Bostonian: "Don't be cross!" The phrase, one of her favorites, dispelled my anger in the past because of its quaint absurdity. But nothing was normal now. My fury at her illness had taken over.

Above and beyond the feelings the doc and the cancer stirred up, new agendas were generated.

Nancy Falk Schifrin Fox, designated patient, wished to be shielded from further negativity of any kind, to be allowed to go at will "to the seashore," an imaginary retreat her mother years ago adapted from a long-forgotten movie. A make-believe world either mom or daughter could inhabit in isolation when life grew problematic.

Nance, designated victim with a life-threatening disease, also wanted to have every whim totally met.

I knew I'd give that my best shot but, as I increasingly transformed into a midlife servant, wondered who'd shore me up? As husband and partner and caregiver, although my life was not threatened, my orderly universe surely was.

Voila, an insight: Belatedly I recognized that two married friends had waited at the hospital during my wife's surgery as much for me as for her. Nance, even while swatting her own demons, had lovingly suggested I might need help.

I was grateful. It would have been rough sitting there alone with my partner's 27-year-old daughter, who had coped by withdrawing emotionally.

Wednesday, Nov. 23

Nancy threw herself into Thanksgiving preparations. She concocted half a dozen traditional courses, ensuring that each guest (and I) could overeat.

Taking into account she'd undergone surgery less than a week ago, Nance's strength and energy levels could be classified as astounding. When asked about it, she said, "I'm thankful I'm alive and able to make dinner for people I love."

Smirking, I replied: "I'm thankful you're alive, too, and able to make dinner for me."

It didn't take long, unfortunately, for giving thanks to give way to picturing a future that makes me as shaky as an Elvis imitator. At 2:45 a.m. I awakened with fever and closed throat, pushed to the brink of upchucking.

I desperately tried to lighten things up. "I'm sick 'cause I need attention," I moaned through a smile I hoped she'd interpret as mostly mischievous.

Thursday, Nov. 24

Dinner went well. Nancy's spunk heartened all six guests. Everyone helped clean up but, dear god of liquid suds and industrial-strength silver polish, we had dirtied an incredible amount of dishes and utensils.

Nance, misty-eyed, later reflected that she "felt very supported. It was perfect, just what I wanted: great friends, family, food, talk." Talk included a vague plan to travel to Greece when the treatments were finished. The idea itself perked us up, allowing us to look beyond the tension and loss of power.

No one conversed directly with Nance about the cancer, though. Unspoken taboo. I was, in contrast, deluged with questions in the living room while she dressed the salad and spooned cranberry sauce onto a plate in the kitchen.

Only one friend, a registered nurse with a hippie past and a mystical bent, didn't need to ask. From experience, she could predict tomorrow.

She'd watched the rollercoaster in motion before.

Friday, Nov. 25

My gargantuan cold knocked the wind out of me as thoroughly as a heavyweight champ's punch might have. But it provided Nancy with a new role — handmaiden to a bedridden husband. Concentrating on my ailment, she declared, was "easier than focusing on the cancer."

The surgeon had predicted we'd be consumed. We hadn't believed him. "We can't let that happen," I'd said to Nance. "We'll have regular lives."

For the time being, at least, we don't.

Some women and caregivers hide their breast-cancer stuff; we're telling everyone in sight about it — so we can vent and they can sympathize.

Sunday, Nov. 27

A sidesplitting Bill Cosby video highlighted a triple-feature comedy weekend. But the balm lasted only as long as the tapes ran; as closing credits rolled, fright rushed back in.

"I know it's hackneyed but I love my wife so much it hurts. Why'd it take almost 30 years to re-discover her if we're to have only a few years? We were supposed to grow old together. I'm scared shitless, God. Please don't let the cancer steal her from me."

Tuesday, Nov. 29

"I work, I see a friend for lunch, I work some more," Nancy said. "Inside, I bounce between hope and fear."

As do many of our friends.

Some insist everything's magically cool; a few stay away, as if Nance had contracted leprosy and were highly contagious; one or two act as if she'll die tomorrow. The vast majority, mercifully, have remained realistic. They know the cancer means six or seven months of treatment hell but anticipate that in the long run she'll be just fine, thank you.

Wednesday, Nov. 30

My wife took "a sensational walk" with Bentley, our rust-colored golden retriever, and an acquaintance. "I revel in the beauty of where I live," she said. "I want to stay alive and be here to take it all in."

Friday, Dec. 2

Shock-time again, precisely two weeks after the first. Pathology results bellowed this afternoon that Nancy's cancer was "aggressive." That meant chemotherapy will be mandatory, along with its side effects — nausea, vomiting, hair loss.

Her oncologist, a striking woman with chiseled white hair and skinny body, will be in charge.

She raced through the details with alarming efficiency.

First came more bad news: "Any cancer cells that have slipped into the bloodstream will not respond to hormone treatment."

So we can cross that out, alone or in combination with the chemo.

But then she wrapped all the goodies we craved in one verbal bundle: "But we're expecting a cure."

She became the first physician I'd heard use that word in connection with the cancer; everyone else had adhered to "remission."

The chemotherapy might be "short and sweet," she added.

Her words came straight from some unwritten "Handbook for Joy." Speak a few sentences the patient and caregiver desperately want to hear. Sprinkle in a phrase or two of tenderness. Instant messiah.

Nance leapt on the joywagon. She proclaimed she was "planning to get through the treatments with minimum discomfort."

Wishful thinking? Maybe. An affirmation? Absolutely.

Regardless, the oncologist used it as a springboard to talk about two patients with an identical chemotherapy regimen. She swore the tale was not apocryphal.

The first allegedly reported, "It's been horrible. I've vomited four times, and sometimes the treatments exhaust me."

The second said, "I'm doing okay. I've only vomited four times, and I only get tired now and then."

On tap for my wife are four doses of chemical poison, three weeks apart, trailed by daily radiation for six to seven weeks (if her whiter-than-white skin can tolerate being scorched). Those protocols will follow Nance's next surgery, to remove two of the three levels of lymph nodes beneath her right arm, which will let lab technicians check if the breast cancer has spread. [In the future, this procedure would change radically, with only sentinel nodes normally being removed, but my partner was years too early to benefit from the advance.]

Possible side effects will be numbness on the underside of the arm, swelling on the top. Odds favor neither being permanent, but nobody's betting.

Worry about the side effects has boosted Nance's fear quotient. She's stirred regularly at 3 a.m., vulnerable, shaking me awake and whispering, "I'm frightened. Please hold me."

Soothing her has required my squeezing like a boa.

"That need is a lot more common than you might expect," noted the oncologist, the second person within days who predicted a metaphoric roll-ercoaster for us. "One day you'll believe Nancy's been cured, the next day you'll think she's going to die."

The cancer specialist became the second part of a four-physician day. I was present for each session. Likewise for all the tests and aftermaths so far.

If I can't be Mr. Fix-it — and I've adjusted to the idea that I can't — I want to be there for her (wherever "there" is) whenever feasible.

First up today, an annual checkup with Nance's "primary-care physician." A touch of irony: He found her in tiptop physical health except for the minor detail that she's been hosting a wicked bunch of malignant cells.

He did give us one worrisome tidbit to munch on.

He recommended that the surgeon examine the sutured breast. A small blood clot apparently had formed beneath Nance's stitches and black-and-blue marks.

The third medic du jour, another oncologist, was a Christopher Walken double with a monotone, slumber-producing voice. Nevertheless, we found him compassionate, attentive and willing to reply in detail. And he had no objections to being relegated to "expert second opinion."

Finally, the surgeon, who in his stock white coat resembled a TV ad for an indigestion remedy, ended our doc-athon by draining some of the clotted blood via a fine-needle aspiration. I squeamishly left the examination room shortly before he broke the skin.

He scheduled another appointment for next week, to duplicate the procedure, and suggested he reopen and clean out the incision, if necessary, when he performed the lymphectomy. "Okay," whimpered Nance, stifling every thought and sensation she could.

Her emotions didn't surface until she punched her thoughts into the computer at bedtime:

"Hearing the words 'aggressive' and 'chemotherapy' were incredibly difficult, my worst dread coming true. This is probably the hardest thing I've ever had to face."

Saturday, Dec. 3

Nancy briefly saw her daughter today and brainwashed herself into believing "she'll be there for me, in spite of all the evidence to the contrary."

She then "hid in the woods of financial responsibility, paying bills to keep myself occupied."

Her anxiety has become more and more conspicuous to me, dangling like a tarnished pendant around her neck. "I'm afraid," she murmured halfway through her chore, "of looking and feeling like a cancer patient, announcing it to the world by my wig, baldness or whatever. And I'm afraid of the treatments."

Even worse, the disease has started to undermine our closeness.

Love can be a panacea, I was taught as a kid. And New Age disciplines underscored that theme for me as an adult "seeker." But the cancer has made us scared our affection may give way like a roof with too many tons of snow on it.

Sunday, Dec. 4

Tonight Nancy turned into a walking wound whose scab had been torn off. The rawness followed our going to a posthumous session of a group that had nurtured a friend whose breast cancer had eaten into her brain.

Nance and I had been caregivers for months and months. We'd been at her bedside seconds before her death, holding her cold hands, gently kissing her bald scalp.

The woman — my funny, bright co-worker and our sensitive, ultra-feminist buddy — had died only four weeks before my wife's disease was diagnosed. In some bizarre way, our frequent visits had prepared us for the courage we need to face Nance's cancer.

Tonight, though, my partner's horror was etched into her eyes. She confessed later that at various points of the memorial "the only things in the room" were herself, her diagnosis and her anxiety.

"I didn't want to be the one the service would be held for in a year," she said.

We talked incessantly about cancer on the way home, and as I cuddled her later in bed. Although it's no longer chewing up her body, the illness is chewing up and spitting out both our lives. Even when we can manage to distract ourselves, an invisible force yanks us back to Cancerland, a concept for a grisly theme park I came up with but would gladly cede to Stephen King.

It might feel like forever to me, yet we've actually been gaping at the cancer gargoyles in our heads for a measly three months — if we're counting the time since Nance found the first lump during one of her regular self-exams.

That one had prompted brooding, lost sleep, an examination by my wife's internist, and a biopsy 10 days later. The diagnosis: fatty tissue. Benign cells had been messing with our minds. "Just keep an eye on it," said a couple of medical pros. We did. And the tumor disappeared without help within weeks.

Nance had found the second mass in October. She and her prime physician agreed to — what else? — "keep an eye on it." When it hadn't shrunk by early November, he referred her to the surgeon, who ordered a mammogram.

The lumpectomy came nine days after that.

All of a sudden, everybody else's fight against breast cancer had become personal. We could even relate to females scaling a faraway peak.

Today's San Francisco Examiner carried a story about next month's assault by 20 breast-cancer survivors on Argentina's 22,835-foot Aconcagua, highest mountain in the Western hemisphere. The climbers, all from Northern California, range from 21 to 68. They seek to raise $2.3 million by selling T-shirts and other souvenirs to elevate hope among Americans with the disease.

The paper quoted a participant: "We're not trying to say that breast-cancer survivors should climb mountains, but they should reclaim their lives."

Easier said than done.

Everything might look bright from a mountaintop but Nance and I've been in a funk that's digging a black hole in our lives. I've started to envy all the women and their mates who've won their battles while we still face ours.

Monday, Dec. 5

We proved last night cancer simply can't rework our marriage: We argued over something trivial.

That's not a rare situation — two only-children lock-stepped into jockeying for position. But Nancy's breast cancer gave me guilt about the bickering.

I dissolved the tension this morning by phoning her from the commuter-ferry terminal. "I'll always be in your corner," I said.

Less than an hour later, I tried to raise the consciousness level at work by prominently displaying the pink "breast-cancer awareness" ribbon I'd gotten at yesterday's memorial.

Tuesday, Dec. 6

Mid-afternoon, Nancy conferred with marketing pros at the San Francisco Zoo, one of her clients. They left her confident the cancer won't destroy her life as a public-relations consultant.

But concurrent support sessions later in the day depleted us both.

Nance exited from hers pondering how she could "possibly be in a group of people with life-threatening diseases? Maybe I'm there to help them as much as they're there to help me."

My group included a woman whose husband died four days ago. Her grief was like an old Ms. Pac-Man game, attacking everyone in sight.

For me, it was a no-brainer that we must immediately learn ways to hop over hurdles like that, and to reduce stress. For sure, we also have to continue shopping for substitute groups that emphasize survival.

Thursday, Dec. 8

Today my partner did "one of the strangest things I've ever done — go to a hands-on healer, because several people recommended him and because I'm terrified of going into tomorrow's surgery and I want everything possible in my arsenal of spiritual, psychological, physical and metaphysical goodies. So I let a perfectly strange man place his warm hands on the lymph nodes that'll be removed.

"The strangest thing was that I never told him what side, but he went to the right without hesitation."

Friday, Dec. 9

A couple of hours before the surgeon began scooping out a batch of Nancy's lymph nodes, her radiologist disclosed she'll get 32 treatments, five per week.

Nance found an "instantaneous rapport with her, and her quirky, humorous yet straightforward New York style." I readily saw why. The doc, a poster child for skinny people, wears a broader and brighter smile than Julia Roberts can muster.

My wife was momentarily put off by the radiologist's declaration that Nance's fair skin "will be a challenge." But she twinkled when the doctor added that she'd successfully "treated an albino."

The good cheer lasted through the lymphectomy, an operation that turned out to be a hitchless but not stitchless procedure. Once defogged, Nance felt the pain of the surgery as well as discomfort from a tube that drained fluids from the incision.

She was optimistic nonetheless. "I seem to be traveling a craggy, twisted pathway that'll lead to renewed health," she proclaimed.

I was happy to concur.

Saturday, Dec. 10

The hospital discharged Nancy mid-morning. Next stop, home for drug-induced bed-rest.

"Woody is wonderful. Friends call, send flowers and gifts. I feel very loved and cared for," she observed in her now-and-then diary. *"I'm also feeling strange as the recipient of all this outpouring. I'm used to being the outpourer, not the outpouree."*

Sunday, Dec. 11

"I can't believe how well I'm feeling," said Nancy.

Between sleeping and resting, resting and sleeping, she phoned a girl-hood-adulthood Detroit friend to arrange The Call to Mother in a couple of days.

Her mom, who'd rushed headlong into her mid-80s with an unneeded cane that gets her sympathy and primo restaurant tables, didn't know about the breast cancer.

I knew, meanwhile, the need to subjugate my life to Nance's and her disease has produced a little antagonism inside me. *"Being a male caregiver may be a deviant state. Maybe women are inherently more nurturing."*

Monday, Dec. 12

My suffering sweetheart tried on scarves, hats and turbans to disguise her upcoming cue-ball look.

Afterward, a female acquaintance brought her an Asian delicacy. My wife designated it as "Thai chicken soup" though it contained neither chicken nor soup. That's become her lighthearted generic label for all gift foods that arrive in the name of good health.

Tuesday, Dec. 13

My wife lived through The Call. She'd orchestrated it so she was armed with the positive surgical results and the assistance of a Detroit friend who'd dropped by her mom's and plied her with a glass of Harvey's Bristol Cream.

Nancy's mom, as predicted, fired a plethora of questions. Uncharacteristically, the octogenarian paid attention to the responses.

Wednesday, Dec. 14

Nancy crashed last night into a barrier of "the most excruciating pain I've experienced since childbirth." She hoped her stomach cramps were "symptomatic only of gas," but sweats and queasiness followed. Moving her legs out of bed became an ordeal.

We raced to our hospital's cancer center, where the physician on duty diagnosed it. "Anxiety. Acute."

The radiologist ran into us in a hallway as we were leaving. She read Nance's still-colorless face and instinctively did something exceptional for a doctor: She hugged my wife. We luxuriated in the moment.

She had missed my partner's private outburst after the intern's quickie diagnosis, though. "I hate it," Nance had whispered to me. "I've been through two surgeries, countless medications, knives, stitches, germs and germ-fighters, chills and a low-grade fever. I don't like being labeled The Woman with Anxiety."

I'd suggested she "try to disregard the anxiety and be thankful you're alive and under treatment."

I could've sworn I heard her snarl.

My own angst directed me to a comparatively new support group for guys whose partners have breast cancer. It promises "a sympathetic forum to discuss the challenge for the man to be supportive and loving."

Thursday, Dec. 15

Hell must be something like this. We get zero chance to catch our breath because of one crisis after another, day after day.

Topping today's list was a visit to a dermatologist who specializes in circumspection and hedging his bets. The rash Nancy had scratched from neck to ankles last night, he theorized, might be a reaction to one drug or another, or a combination of them. "Or maybe it was something you ate."

Nance couldn't care less what created the problem; she simply wanted it to go away. "He smothered me in prednisone, but I still itch," she grumbled as we left his office.

Friday, Dec. 16

Like an attentive plumber, the surgeon checked Nancy's drain. "It'll come out next week," he said.

Said she, "I won't miss it."

She also won't miss another support group she tried. She'd sat next to a woman who is battling cancer after having survived a father's Satanic cult rituals and incestuous bent.

My mate had remained motionless until her turn to speak. Then she'd said, "I'm Nancy Fox and I just have breast cancer."

Saturday, Dec. 17

My wife, a self-anointed detective on a comprehensive search for the perfect wig, was delighted to find a style and color that pleased us both. But she didn't order it. Her reluctance, I surmised, was partially because it was inordinately expensive.

The prospect of losing her hair ("my favorite thing on my head") has continued to unsettle her. "It'll grow back," she's said repeatedly, apparently struggling to convince herself.

My mantra, spoken to her again and again, is that I'll love her bald. She doesn't believe me.

I do.

Monday, Dec. 19

When the surgeon removed the long tubing that let cloudy fluids flow out of Nancy's incision, my wife, relieved, twirled like a toddler in a recital and parodied a "Wizard of Oz" lyric: "I no longer have a drain."

Tuesday, Dec. 20

Nancy wants deeper camaraderie with females, the gender with breasts. Not surprising.

Thursday, Dec. 22

The dentist cleaned and rinsed my partner's teeth. Then he flooded her with information about the expected softening of her gums from the chemo.

Saturday, Dec. 24

Nancy and I re-hung paintings. Switching them from room to room became a cheap-thrills way of altering our environment and dodging cancer thoughts. We had fun.

Now there's a word we've under-used lately.

Sunday, Dec. 25

We overcame our resistance and screened a video that featured women talking about their breast cancer. Nancy decided it was "reassuring they're all doing well and that there are so many others in the same boat as we are."

The documentary did buoy us, particularly after our skirmish late last night. I'd exploded because of a series of minor incidents in which she'd wiped me out. "You're selfish, thoughtless and inattentive to me," I'd yelled.

"You're inflexible," she'd lashed back.

We'd become, once again, two tots in a sandbox tossing crud at each other.

After we'd made up, Nance said, "I hate it when I invisibilize and hurt you." But I ended up guilt-ridden because, no matter how justified my anger, I'd tongue-lashed a breast-cancer patient.

Tuesday, Dec. 27

Nancy experimented with guided imagery today.

During the visualization, Red Riding Hood, whom she selected as a fantasy protector, "winked at, flirted with and mooned the wolf, which represented the cancer."

The creature slinked into the woods after being confronted, and my wife spun around in a diaphanous white dress spotlighted by the sun that poured through the treetops. She held a white and gold crystal in her hand.

Afterward, she felt exhilarated.

I, too, felt marvelous — due to her delight and to my annual physical, which put my heart rate, blood pressure and electrocardiogram readings in the "normal" range.

Wednesday, Dec. 28

Nancy tried yet another women's group. "It was the best so far, but I still haven't found a perfect match," she declared.

"Just keep looking. You'll find the right one," I replied, more as encouragement than an expression of honest belief.

In recent days, I've thought a lot about support — and about doctors. I've pondered how they too often take the advice of sales reps from pharmaceutical houses.

Being a Libra and always looking for balance, I've also considered how most docs work hard and are on call at all hours, and how they're often the one-eyed in the land of the blind.

4

SUPPORT

The instant a cancer diagnosis takes place, going it alone vanishes as a viable option — for either the patient or caregiving partner. But the big question is where to find appropriate assistance and support.

For Nancy and me, the basic order was a no-brainer.

First came the healing professionals — Western medicine, then Eastern, then holistic (with an emphasis on visualizations, which several of her healers had recommended). We leaned on them all, to rid her body of the cancer and to keep the disease from returning.

We didn't give an ant's ass what worked, just that something did.

Even as the pros labored to repair her flesh, we sought others to soothe our minds. Friends helped. So, to a lesser extent, did family. Psychiatry unlocked an issue or two. And lastly, after lengthy trial-and-error searches, we separately joined fledgling, single-gender support groups.

Along with that multitude of safety nets came an avalanche of reading materials — books, magazine and newspaper articles, endless online bits and pieces.

Learn and discard. Absorb and block. Siphon out unnecessary information.

Learn each person is an individual, not a statistic.

Learn breast cancer couldn't care less about race, creed, color or politics: It is the most common cancer among Israelis and Palestinians living in Gaza and the West Bank.

Learn there will be rough "I'm-all-alone-and-nobody-understands-what-I'm-going-through" times regardless of how much support you gather. (To offset those bad periods, learn you can find ways to illuminate the dark alleys of your brain so you can stay in the here-and-now and stop worrying about tomorrow.)

Yet no matter how bright a breast cancer patient's outlook (or a male caregiver's), fear and thoughts of loss may morph into a gargantuan ogre.

And sessions of my Marin Man to Man group, which mainly tilt toward the optimistic and constructive, still occasionally stir up feelings guys would rather not confront.

We've never been able, for example, to make the primary breast cancer bogeyman — recurrence — evaporate completely.

Death fears also drop in on our Wednesday morning sessions — infrequently, thank heavens. But it can be outright dispiriting that we sometimes digest such factoids as breast cancer having killed 339,000 American women during the Vietnam War while 59,000 Americans died in the conflict.

Nor was it easy when a dropout from the group, a sailor, phoned me from Florida. He'd fled there to clear his head after his wife booted him out.

I comforted him, temporarily. But she died only a few weeks later, the first fatality connected to Man to Man. There was no apparent medical reason for her demise.

"It was as if she pushed me and everybody else of importance out of her life so she could let go," he subsequently lamented.

Though the group as a whole saw that as a highly atypical circumstance, for the next couple of months attendees struggled to keep conversations airy and detached. No one admitted projecting himself into the widower's place, but we all did it. My own anxiety lit up like a flare on a moonless night.

Eventually, optimism prevailed again.

"We don't talk about it much, but there's pride in our very existence," one member observed, "especially since there's so damned little support for male caregivers anywhere on the planet."

His opinion mirrored that of most who joined us, regardless of whether they became regular eat-and-talkers or visited only once. Many, to be sure, initially checked out Man to Man not because they thought they needed shoring up, but as a result of their partners' nagging.

Nance, of course, was *my* prompter — partially because she was pre-occupied with her own situation.

On an early Man to Man website, she explained her motivation: "Since my bout with cancer sucked up all of my energy, physically and psychologically, I know I was not 'available' in many ways to comfort my husband, a role I generally assume as his wife.

"I was too scared, hurting, focused on my own healing, schedules, aches and pains to deal with 'how it was for him.' I just wanted him to be there. And he was.

"I should have known he was equally frightened, but I didn't. I should have known he needed to talk about it, but I was the wrong audience. I should have been able to be there for his concerns, but I wasn't. I was too wrapped up in my own.

"There were even times when he accompanied me to my treatments that I wished he weren't there. I didn't want him to see it. I didn't want to worry about his reactions to what was going on. And I couldn't even tell him that at the time, because I didn't want to hurt him, since he was being so sweet and loving.

"So when we found out about Marin Man to Man, I was thrilled. A place to vent with 'the guys.' A place for him to articulate all the stuff that was swirling around in his introspective head."

Articulate I did.

I enjoyed being able to say that "the pure necessity of living one day at a time" helped me focus. And that I needed to set practical goals — like cleaning up after dinner every night even when weary.

I also relished simply being able to confide in the men ("Nance was big-time bitchy last night").

They accepted an outburst such as that as a fleeting perspective, a manifestation of my inner scaredy-cat. They knew I treasured my wife yet found the rollercoaster too difficult to handle that particular minute.

And I knew they knew tiny gripes could pop up anytime — despite data that support-group members generally fare better than those who meander the cancer landscape solo.

Nance, in her journal, habitually voiced thanks for not having to go through everything unaccompanied. She savored the benefit of receiving metaphoric shots in the arm from a substantial network of associates and by, above all, having me at her side.

But being her principal caregiver could be extremely draining.

It came as no surprise, then, that a report from the American Society of Clinical Oncology indicated clinical depression might result from the "mental beating" partners of cancer survivors took while their loved ones battled the illness.

A main researcher had deduced that spouses and other caregivers experienced "similar emotional and greater social long-term costs of cancer than survivors."

A few years back, a small Danish study screamed that male partners of breast cancer patients were 39 percent more apt to be hospitalized for mood disorders such as anxiety and depression than men who didn't face caregiving issues.

Two years after that, an Ohio State University study underscored the problem.

It showed breast cancer caregivers riddled with guilt, depression and fear of loss were likely to get headaches and stomach pain, and have weaker immune responses.

Somewhere along the way I learned that taking care of myself had to be a priority if I were to be an effective partner.

And that meant ensuring that I'd get help and support from friends and co-workers to force me to leave the house, and, therefore, get away from both tension and partner (if only for a few minutes), and that I'd eat and sleep well, exercise, meditate, and do selfish things I especially enjoyed.

Considering our dual and individual stress, it didn't shock us that regardless how hard Nance or I wanted to shut them out, repugnant thoughts, with all the charisma of banana slugs, periodically invaded our fragile minds.

Happily, we — and most patients and caregivers — could rebuff them more often than not with life-affirming memories.

So both of us clung to each success story, even if it seemed surreal.

One Man to Man colleague reported his wife was "in complete remission, cancer-free after six months as a complete vegetarian, a vegan." Before the diet, she'd been diagnosed with breast cancer that had spread to her spinal column. We'd all presumed she was in deep trouble, and were elated by the change.

But her improvement prompted her husband to try what most guys deemed extreme — a wheat-grass diet that "features daily implants of the grain's juice through a catheter inserted into the colon, daily oral doses of the juice, and daily enemas or colonics."

Our group split equally between "ugh!" and "yechh!" But the enema advocate was on Cloud Nine that his regimen was helping.

Another chap, years later, purged himself with a three-week regimen of steamed veggies — followed, shortly thereafter, with a 10-day fast in which he consumed only lemonade laced with a dab of maple syrup and a sprinkle of paprika.

Along with the toxins, he lost 45 pounds.

As a group, we voiced unanimity that each of us should "do his own thing" health-wise, whatever that entailed, but also agreed we must beware of "excessive sacrifice."

That specific group-think stemmed from my telling about Nance joining me at an Indian restaurant and ordering spicy food she didn't like in an attempt "to do something nice" to repay my caregiving. She'd gotten really sick the next day, so neither of us ending up feeling good about her offering.

It was decidedly more positive attending a 50th birthday party for a wife in her support group.

The woman's middle-aged confederates rallied like squealing cheerleaders at a high-school playoff game. Their tagalong male partners, forewarned that jubilation was mandatory, obediently displayed signs of euphoria.

Hors d'oeuvres, dinner and cocktail twaddle each earned a passing grade, but the restaurant's incomparable dance-floor energy was what captivated our crowd. Celebrants acted as gleeful as if an estranged relative had hit a $100 million lottery and divided it.

We jiggled to rock 'n' roll from the '50s, '60s and '70s, ignoring how clumsy — or dated — we may have appeared to bartenders, servers and other diners.

In truth, none of the participants might ever totally purge recollections of slogging through breast cancer and its perpetual treatments. But for hours that night, we mid-lifers unloaded the old horrors by twitching like dogs shaking off bathwater.

Unfortunately, the change from gloomy to giddy, from morose to mindless, didn't happen nearly as often as any of us would have liked. Many members of Nance's support group — and mine, too — often experienced low laugh-ometer ratings.

Because of that tendency, caregivers and patients seemed to clutch onto every moment of levity, even teeny or forced ones.

One woman yanked off her wig in public after her husband had been playfully tugging on its French braid. He couldn't help cackling nervously. "It was the first time I'd laughed in a long while," he reported.

Giggles, titters and full belly-laughs were evoked by a prosthesis peddler displaying a variety of wares to Nance's cohorts. Samples ranged from plain bra fillers and fake boobs to bogus nipples. Grinning like pubescent schoolgirls, the women merrily swapped items, compared sizes and colors, and tried on lines of matching and non-matching breast "accessories."

Many also found amusement through hair-replacement, baldness having let them live out some "grass-is-greener" daydreams.

Former proud possessors of long, straight hair opted for naturally curly wigs — and vice versa. Women afraid to dip into bottles of bleach or dye or rinse slipped easily into new looks and, with them, an ephemeral personality transplant.

One guy later recounted an incident in which his wife "owned one bandana/hair number that was so different that, when we went to the airport, our son walked right by without a hint of who she was. She had to walk alongside him and bump him once or twice before he had a clue."

If life for Nance and me couldn't continually be a barrelful of amusement, we did realize we merely had to shift an attitude, change how we perceived the world around us.

From my memory bank comes a pair of for-instances.

While strolling in downtown San Francisco, I'd often seen despair on the faces of the homeless who slouched in doorways, a ragged army battling against starvation and exposure. I'd grimaced when a tourist tried to shake off his discomfort by flippantly referring to them as "residentially challenged."

One rainy morning a group of pedestrians was approached by an old, old African American caressing a red blanket so ratty that Linus would have trashed it in a microsecond. The beggar evoked a sunnier impression — spurring the tourists to dig into their pockets or purses — with a one-liner: "Can you help this very young Jewish boy work his way through college?"

Another chilly day I neared a sullen, craggy-faced moocher with dark matted hair that smelled as if it hadn't been washed in months. He sat cross-legged behind a tin cup. I was certain his demeanor came from his need to panhandle.

A closer look, however, revealed the source of his dismay was the falling stock market prices he was perusing in that morning's Wall Street Journal.

First-timers at Man to Man meetings likewise were apt to make erroneous presumptions.

One of our earliest members wrote about it for our website: "My initial hesitation proved to be completely unwarranted. This wasn't the TV sitcom style group-therapy session I dreaded; no one was going to ask, 'And how does that make you feel?'

"Instead, it was a group of guys who were (or had been) in the same place I was, complete with all of the unknowns, frustrations, worries, etc. It was a place to ask questions, get answers to questions I hadn't thought to ask, and find comfort in the realization that what I was experiencing was no different than what everyone else was going through."

The truth is, the fellows prefer chatting about ordinary, non-cancer subjects.

We've been known to gab about auto repairs and fix-it projects, the weather, computers, the size of mosquitoes, vacations, buffets, politics, dogs, motorcycles, religion, five-legged cows and jobs. Contrary to other men's groups, perhaps, sports rarely make it onto our agenda.

From time to time, we've temporarily expanded Man to Man's parameters upon request.

A guy who himself had had breast cancer joined us, teaching that awareness levels stay low because fewer than 2,000 cases are diagnosed annually.

A handful of men whose partners had other cancers also attended for a while. We figured we might not be able to advise about medications or treatments in those instances, but we'd all become sensitive, lay experts — to one degree or another — in psychology, feelings and emotions.

Breast cancer, of course, has always remained Topic A — whenever anyone wants to talk about it.

Should I ever become frustrated that more men don't seek the help they obviously need, or that some give us only a single-shot trial, these words from a Marin Man to Man organizer who handed me the reins almost two decades ago reassure me:

"Those who drop in and don't come back," he'd said wisely, "take whatever they need and get support elsewhere."

A year after her final treatment, though thrilled with the level of support that enveloped her, Nance still had trouble expressing her innermost feelings sometimes — especially her anger at the disease and at me for being healthy.

And she still felt guilty about needing me to watch over her.

When she had to ask for help, she'd cite an instance when she'd taken care of me, as if that had earned her credits.

As for my own frequently suppressed rage, I once let it loose when we were going over papers for insurance reimbursements, a pile we'd let slide for months because our priorities were elsewhere. Insurance companies, so profitably calculating and cold and geographically far away, made wonderful targets for our misplaced wrath.

In spite of her reluctance to probe many negative feelings since the diagnosis, Nance — at my request — listed some of the low points:

"Hearing the words 'It's cancer.'

"Facing chemotherapy.

"Feeling the chunk of hair fall out of my head and knowing the rest was coming out right behind it, exactly on schedule.

"Being scared.

"Knowing how poorly and sickly and old I looked no matter how hard I tried to make it better.

"*Going to endless doctors for endless exams and endless treatments.*
"*Having dozens of hands punch and probe my breast.*"

She was less resistant to count off some major highs:
"*The first time I went out without a hat on in short, short hair.*
"*Being able to stay up a whole day without napping.*
"*Having everyone help me.*
"*Realizing there were many things I could do to feel better and to heal —
and doing them.*"

She then gave herself new objectives, including filling her life — in the
moment — with yesses.

"*I know I have a propensity for saying no, and I am trying very hard to say
yes, to look for the good, the possible, the positive.*

"*It's been, it is, a challenging road, partially because of the cancer, partially
because I'm in my middle age and am facing all of the issues surrounding that
time.*

"*I can be happy and healthy. I deserve it. I've worked hard. As a card-carrying member of the Cancer Club, a card-carrying member of the human race,
I want joy in the years I have to spend here. At my age, there are probably less
of them in front of me than there are behind. That's okay, though. I've come to
peace with it.*"

While reading that journal entry, I realized I hadn't quite reached such
a tranquil state yet. But I was pretty sure my peace with the aging process
and breast cancer was likely to show up exponentially faster than, to use a
slightly over-the-top example, a lasting peace in the Middle East.

5

CHEMOTHERAPY

During Nancy's cancer treatments, staying positive was as difficult as accepting the reality of suicidal fanatics intentionally crashing jets into World Trade Center and Pentagon buildings on Sept. 11, 2001. Terrorism on U.S. soil. Cancer-terrorism in Nance's body. Both were unthinkable at first. Both would change our worlds at the core, remind us to cherish every day. These journal extracts underscore our successes and failures — and plainly indicate the volatility of our lives.

Thursday, Dec. 29

Nancy underwent her first chemotherapy treatment today. That started the second stage of the predicted "slash, poison and burn" treatments.

The chemo wasn't physically painful yet my wife felt as if the rug had been snatched from beneath her. She couldn't stop thinking about the toxins dripping into her veins.

Despite my lovingly pressing her hand, the chemo room overlooking a mountain and egrets gliding by the picture window, her headset lulling her with the sounds of a relaxation tape, the special crystal clutched in her hand and the nurses being as soothing as a Frank Sinatra ballad, Nance called it "the hardest day I've ever had in my life."

It wasn't my easiest either.

I felt as if a professional kickboxer had launched a full-strength attack on my stomach.

The session lasted three hours, counting the paperwork and questions, an electrocardiogram, a drug orientation and, as a socko finish, the chemo.

Immediately after she was done taking in the intravenous poisons, we drove to a shop where my red-haired wife — desperate to buy a hairpiece before her tresses start falling out in chunks — picked out a wiglet with a lot of blonde in it.

Then, in quick succession, she experienced chills, fever and nausea.

Friday, Dec. 30

A close friend stayed with Nancy most of the day, serving homemade soup and large bowls of sympathy. My wife felt unexpectedly good.

I experienced a healthy "dose of good," too, after skimming a thin booklet titled "Straight Talk About Breast Cancer," written in part by Dr. Suzanne W. Braddock, a breast cancer patient. My internist, himself a cancer expert, had lent it to me. He claimed it was more in touch with the feelings of patients and their families than most.

The paperback reassured me because I could relate to its common themes. I also found it less difficult to read than pamphlets from agencies that concentrated on worst-case scenarios and scared the bejesus out of us.

One section leapt out.

It said finding a lone cancer cell in the lymph nodes can be equated to finding none at all. And since a single villainous cell was what the experts had discovered in the multiple nodes removed from Nance's body, the information calmed us.

"Straight Talk" was peppered with relevant, usually inspirational quotes. But one we especially related to touched on the awkwardness of friends and clan: "Some people don't know what to do, and they unintentionally say the wrong things. For example, telling someone with cancer not to worry is like telling someone not to breathe. My own mother said to me, 'If you have to have cancer, this is the best kind to have.' I guess people just don't think.'"

My worry of uttering the wrong thing — or of Nance peeking at my journal and misinterpreting a word or phrase and, thus, being hurt or scared — has consistently gnawed at me.

Concurrently, I've grown increasingly frustrated by the unbalanced amount of self-help and other material available for breast cancer patients (tons and tons) compared to that aimed at males or caregivers in general (ounces).

Sunday, Jan. 1

We rested, fatigued emotionally and physically.

<u>Monday, Jan. 2</u>

Nancy, downplaying her emotional anguish, claimed "for the first time since I've been dealing with this illness, I've become depressed, cranky and out of sorts." Hocus, pocus! By waving a mental wand she magically dissolved her numerous bad days since the cancer's onset.

"'Perky' wouldn't be an apt description of my temperament today," she continued. "I was 'grumpy.'"

In truth, Nance has assumed at various times since the diagnosis the persona of each of Disney's seven animated dwarfs — Grumpy, Dopey, Sleepy, Sneezy, Bashful, Happy and Doc.

And at Macy's, where my wife prospected today for new pajamas, she became an eighth little person — Spiteful.

I had the audacity to say no to something she wanted. Then, when I objected to her follow-up rant, she ridiculed me in singsong fashion. My irate inner brat kicked in, to battle hers, and unleashed a tactic my wife considers the ultimate sin: I raised my voice.

The verbal warfare escalated on the way to the drugstore to refill two prescriptions. When she threatened to walk home, an uphill trek I knew would sap her already skimpy energy, I completely lost it. I recklessly shouted that she should "get a fucking nurse and I'll move out."

Summoning all her theatricality, Nance responded by scrawling what I said on a scrap of paper. It would be permanent proof of my indiscretion.

Then my spouse, an expert at altering reality to fit the way she wants it to be, went the extra mile — she scribbled a phrase I had not uttered: "I won't be there when you lose your hair."

Her revisionism was revealing. She saw, when I later pointed to what she'd written, that her dread of going bald had leapt off the charts. Just before turning out the lights she recalled that as a girl with braids down to her waist, she'd panicked when her mother demanded she cut them off.

Though I sympathized with her daymare, I came to bed furious. My anger had puffed up because Nance had used me as a foil when her demons showed themselves.

But she'd also poured fuel on my pyre by disclosing she's been taking Prozac since the cancer diagnosis.

Because I'm a communications nut, her tiny lies of omission have driven me bonkers for years. She'd typically say she "just forgot" to tell me. This time, for a change, she admitted her secret was intentional. She was afraid I'd object.

The incident made me want to run away.

<u>Wednesday, Jan. 4</u>

A new friend visited Nancy, bringing compassion, buffoonery and anecdotes. Later, a couple of old female pals helped her evening speed by and presented an opportunity for me to dine out with a buddy.

Her summation: "It was a good day."

My assessment differed. Sex — or, more accurately, a diminishing frequency — has begun to unnerve me. I'll bet the idea hasn't crossed her mind any more often in recent weeks than an impending invasion of Venusians.

<u>Tuesday, Jan. 10</u>

Nancy asked an acupuncturist-herbalist to add traditional Chinese medicine to her regimen of Western treatment. I'm unsure of my reaction.

Nance's hair, meanwhile, came into focus as clearly as a follicle under a microscope. Tufts began falling out this morning, exactly a dozen days after her first chemo — as advertised. She held the first cluster in her hand at 3 a.m.

"It's really hard to deal with this," she said tearfully.

I hastily wrote words that cheered her. She read them over and over:

"Woody loves me no matter what.

"So do all the people who surround me.

"This is only temporary.

"My hair will grow back.

"I've chosen to lose my hair rather than my life.

"My beauty is inside, not outside.

"I've prepared by buying a wiglet and other head-coverings.

"I'm not the first, nor the last, to go through this; there are millions of others who have survived cancer and chemo."

Her eyes watered up, she smiled, and then she added a few phrases of her own:

"I'm strong enough to do this.

"I'll find the humor and the fun in this temporary situation.

"God will guide me through.

"I am healing.

"Advantages of having no hair:

"I'll have a few dandruff-free months.

"I'll save money on shampoo and beauty parlors.

"I'll learn from this experience."

"This is still hard," she said, once again tearfully, when she stopped writing. "Really hard."

Wednesday, Jan. 11

Nancy's latest visualization evoked hundreds of "psychiatric-sanitary workers."

Every time they saw a cancer cell, she reported, they "put a plunger on it and dumped it into a wheelbarrow, which they carted out of my body. My body was completely cleansed."

In conjunction with that healing technique, she turned "proactive" into the day's operative word. She couldn't face hair loss cluster by cluster so she, her daughter and I traipsed to the apartment of a hairdresser. Within minutes, the pro had snipped every strand of my mate's long red hair to about a quarter-inch.

"I look like a combination of Mr. Clean and Granny Goose," said Nance. "I can't believe it's me."

Thursday, Jan. 12

My wife wore her wiglet and a hat to a meeting about fundraising for the zoo, one of her clients. Committee members, surprised when she mentioned she had breast cancer, had thought the hair was hers. They expressed confidence she'd continue to work on the event. "I hope that's true," she said to me in private.

Pursuing the positive, Nancy agreed to my request to photograph her with buzz-cut, pajama top and "convict numbers" we'd printed from the computer. Someday, hopefully, we'll compare the photo with her grown-in tresses and chuckle.

For a negligible amount of time, she relaxed and hammed it up, adopting a sultry look and slipping the pajama top off her shoulder.

I do wish she could consistently see herself as I do, as a beautiful creature with or without hair.

Friday, Jan. 13

Nancy spent hours futilely trying to work. "Concentration's a lost cause," she said.

She couldn't even bring herself to play the piano, a love she'd embraced since the age of 3.

She knew exactly where she wanted her git-up-'n'-go to go, but her gas pedal kept jamming. To keep from seeing herself as a petrified driver certain to crash into a mental medial strip, she tried on hats and scarves, listened to tapes about breast cancer, watched videos about the disease, and read and read and read about her illness until her eyes burned.

Sunday, Jan. 15

Chemo-fatigue grabbed control today. Nancy slept nearly all day long.

She did sustain consciousness for dinner with two friends. And she later managed to keep her eyelids open for sex. Although the vaginal dryness was markedly worse than before the chemo, she's been inserting tons of Replens so her vagina does not — contrary to what Nance had impishly prognosticated — "dry up, crack and fall on the floor."

For the third or fourth time in her sleep, however, she experienced leg spasms while curled next to my body afterwards. It rattled me.

My dream about her dying spooked me even more.

I didn't tell her. But it scared me awake and I couldn't shake it off, couldn't sleep again.

Monday, Jan. 16

Nancy joined a Kaiser Permanente support group.

"The women were open," she said, noting it felt like a fitting end to her elongated search. "They're all fighters, every one, and it's good to be among them."

But she wasn't up to battling frigid weather, rain and her cold a second time in one day. So she played hooky from a chi gung class that's teaching her to channel the body's energy for purposes of healing.

For the time being, to help Nance's body heal and to keep mine upright as well, the Bulletin's associate publisher has organized a rotating "food brigade." Various staffers will supply a meal or two each Monday. That's spectacular, because I find 6:45 p.m., when I usually get home, late to start cooking. On second thought, that sentence is a self-serving distortion: The time doesn't matter; I have no big interest in cooking at any hour. Nance by then has curled up in bed anyway, like a glob of candle wax that melted down in a blackout.

Tuesday, Jan. 17

The surgeon, after a routine checkup, affirmed Nancy was "doing well."

My wife then visited her psychiatrist for her first 50-minute hour since the diagnosis. They probed her relationships with her disease and her intimates, me in particular — and the fact that we've begun separating now from then with a B.C. designation: "Before Cancer."

In the evening, I lit a candle in memory of my father, acknowledging aloud how much I miss him. My eyes still water every time I think about his death from prostate cancer 11 years ago.

The commemoration also forced me to ponder other losses in my life: my mom, my grandparents, a woman I lived with in Philadelphia, a close friend, two first-cousins who died in their teens, an aunt, an uncle, and one of Nance's aunts. All told, death in double digits — more than enough for any lifetime.

"Enough. Please, God, enough."

Thursday, Jan. 19

Chemo treatment No. 2.

I again accompanied Nancy into what I've dubbed The Poison Palace. By design we've been able to schedule all Nance's chemotherapy sessions for my lightest workload days.

"It's reassuring to have you with me," emphasized my wife.

Knowing what to expect, we found ourselves considerably less nervous than the first time. And Nance controlled her bout with nausea by sliding an Ativan tablet under her tongue.

This evening, for the first time, during one of the escapist videos we later watched, I kissed the baldness of Nance's head. I was shocked to see myself pull back. It wasn't because she was repulsive in any way but because I'd flashed on my deceased friend and coworker. I immediately had to re-program my brain:

"Your friend was dying; Nance's not."

Friday, Jan. 20

I encouraged Nancy to have five female friends drop in. They staggered their visits in two-hour shifts so the post-chemo duty wouldn't strain any individual. "It was very nourishing, relaxing," my partner reported.

All five road-tested her latest acquisition, a full-length, mostly blonde wig. "It may not be you but it's a fantastic change," opined one. "You look too different," said another.

I presumed Nance would return it and keep searching. It seemed clear, oh goddess of groan-inducing puns, that her dome wasn't going to be re-built in a day.

Saturday, Jan. 21

Tension between Nancy and me has become as thick as bubble wrap.

She objected today to being "supervised and having my every thought and action edited, even when you do it out of love for me." Decoded, I expect that means, "Be close by when I want you here; be anywhere else when I don't."

My problem, invariably, has become how to read her mind to determine exactly when to do what.

Her nastiness quotient has seemed to self-inflate more each month, like a kid gone berserk with an automatic pump and helium balloons. She's often denied being angry about the cancer but, in lieu of lashing out at the disease, has been scapegoating me with scalpel precision. If I'd leave the room to avoid an argument, she'd relentlessly follow. It's as if she were demanding a victim of her own so she wouldn't have to be one.

Monday, Jan. 23

Nancy said her support group "is becoming more valuable as I get to know the women and they get to know me. The level of trust is extraordinary, and the vulnerability that comes about because of the cancer creates a unique and close bond almost instantaneously."

That echoed my thoughts about the men's group.

Tuesday, Jan. 24

My partner and I attended a "Journey to Healing" lecture this evening, purportedly about emotions and communication. We absorbed nothing new. We did, however, find a Marin General social worker cum therapist who agreed to see us as a couple.

Counseling has become a necessity — to deal with our sexuality if nothing else.

Thursday, Jan. 26

As spent as a couple of rock stars at the end of a whirlwind 43-city tour, we fell asleep last night at a reasonable hour. But we were jolted awake by the frenetic pawing of our golden retriever, who was freaked out by the rain and wind and lightning. I calmed him. Nancy couldn't since we both worry he'll accidentally break her skin, which could lead to a treacherous infection. Our concern stemmed from the chemo having severely lowered her white blood cell count and quashed her immune system.

While stroking the pooch until almost dawn, I watched the clock's second-hand move in slo-mo.

I resembled a zombie at work today.

Friday, Jan. 27

We'd seen signs in doctors' offices and hospitals that read, "No perfume, please." We didn't fully understand. But this evening Nancy had a problem with a friend's fragrance — the first time one had nauseated her since the chemo began.

The gal-pal covered her head with a scarf. She also moved as far from Nance as possible and still remain in our living room.

Saturday, Jan. 28

Increasingly, Nancy's become an unhappy camper. "It takes me almost two hours now to get dressed, take pills, stretch my arm in the shower to heal from the latest surgery, put on makeup, scarves, et cetera, et cetera, et cetera," she groaned. "I sometimes don't even want to bother."

On top of that, she's grown furious at being unable to shake the cold and cough that have hung on for two months like a toddler clinging to his mother's dress.

She's also been frustrated having to swim upstream every day against a tidal wave of details that clutter our lives. "Things are slipping through the cracks when I get tired or forgetful," she said sadly.

I couldn't reply that I'd take care of it. She'd sulk if I did. To her, that would prove she's not capable.

Although stress and anxiety have become the top logs on her emotional bonfire, she's by no means the only emotional cripple in our home. For the first time since the diagnosis, I totally broke down today.

I sobbed into her robe as the designated patient turned the tables, stroking my hair and back and assuring me that everything will be okay.

By and large, she can't breathe easily enough to be any sort of caregiver — she has to deal with far too many side effects. Her headaches have grown stronger, and last longer. Her sciatica, in both legs, has become a frequent presence. Fatigue has positioned itself as the meanest enemy.

I've long maintained that when this trial is over, we'll adopt the maxim that "living well is the best revenge." Right now, that seems like hogwash, a hope against hope.

Too often, panic nibbles at me.

It certainly alarmed me this morning to notice her eyes were ringed with black. Every time I've seen similar facial discoloring, it signaled death lurking. I gasped and asked Nance to check with her doctor.

Clergymen have insisted that God gives us nothing we can't handle; they certainly have more faith in Him at this moment than I do.

Sunday, Jan. 29

"I'm sick of being sick," Nancy said this morning.

She's also grown weary of chit-chatting about the disease ("I know my mother will call today, as she does daily, and I don't want to talk to her. The conversations are so repetitive").

I, on the other hand, have loosened up, mainly because the circles around Nance's eyes have faded. It might have been tiredness, or eye make-up she didn't totally remove. Whatever the reason, like rhythm 'n' blues singer James Brown, I felt goooooooooood.

Wednesday, Feb. 1

Hooray, Nancy's no longer housebound despite her immune system having been weakened by the treatments. Doctors advised she could "risk going a movie matinee where there aren't crowds of people," she told me with a look of pure bliss.

"Escape!" instantaneously became our banner.

Getting un-negative can happen that swiftly, but staying positive has become a deliberate, more ragged process.

At Man to Man this morning, an oldtimer moaned that his wife still gets unnerved "every time she feels a new pain, any little pain." Her anxieties have remained constant — that the cancer has recurred — though she's long beyond her final treatment.

The shaky picture caused me to evaluate my own mental status.

I saw I was apt to bounce from joy to despair without missing a beat. Too often sleep-deprived, I've grown grouchier with the passage of each month. And currently, I'm as testy as a rooster in a chicken-less barnyard.

Friday, Feb. 3

Each morning Nancy can reinvent herself. "Will I be a gypsy with scarf and long earrings? Barbra Streisand with a longish pageboy? Or Dorothy Lamour with a dramatic black hat?"

This go-round she chose to be a Streisand clone for lunch with her daughter. "I was very happy to be out," she said.

While Nance was focusing on "out," I had to cope one more time with an "in" — in-somnia. Prodded awake by 4 a.m. dream-state snakes, scorpions and spiders, I toiled at my desk for two hours prior to heading for a scheduled shrink appointment.

Just before leaving I picked up "Straight Talk" and re-read a section titled "What Husbands Can Do To Help Their Wives."

"Tell her you love her. Hug her daily. Fix meals when she's having radiation or chemotherapy treatment. Clean or have someone clean the house. Listen to her fears rather than simply reassuring her everything will be okay. Realize you don't need to be in control, you just need to be there for her. Tell her she's pretty. Do something nice for yourself. Take her for a walk and hold her hand. Check the refrigerator and get the milk, eggs and bread before they run out...Set goals together."

Sound advice.

And it felt awesome that I'd instinctively been doing all of it, including the formidable meal-fixing, before reading the passage.

Saturday, Feb. 4

Two friends brought a tasty soup and delightful anecdotes. One of them, a breast cancer survivor, also brought something exceptional.

She wasted no words. "I've decorated my mastectomy scar. Do you want to see it?"

"Okay," I said, slightly uneasy but trying to be a good sport.

So she flashed us.

Though no fan of the craft, I judged her tattoo to be one of the most beautiful images I'd ever seen. The lengthy pink rose and green vine completely masked the scar tissue. She'd transformed her missing left breast into an art piece.

Sunday, Feb. 5

A visit by Nancy's daughter and her boyfriend quickly pushed my wife into a depression. They stayed for about a minute and a quarter. She apparently felt the need to show up for an obligatory timeframe but the cancer arguably got too scary again.

Monday, Feb. 6

I've maintained an optimistic facade most of the time without any trouble. But I've found it horrific not to freely share my uncertainties with my wife. Instead, the fears have adhered to me like a wad of kid's gum to a theater seat. Breast cancer's most hideous victory may yet turn out to be blocking us from shooting the breeze without self-editing.

Tuesday, Feb. 7

Inevitability can be a heavy leg-iron for my wife.

Losing the locks on her head has been a foregone conclusion. But her body hair has been thinning fast as well. We can no longer deny it's all likely to dwindle into nothingness — eyebrows, eyelashes, pubic hair.

Thursday, Feb. 9

Chemo treatment No. 3.

Nancy's process, in spite of the discomfort, has become "routine." Oncologist exam. Blood test. Errands. Escape into sleep (while moaning about a severe headache).

No nausea, thank goodness.

I hung by her side, as before, through the entire process.

Today's post-treatment errands included making a bank deposit, selecting a romantic-comedy video, and buying treats. A store minutes away from the hospital beckoned to us, a calorie trap waiting to spring. I rang up a pound of cashews, a chunk of chocolate, and a few bags of figs and dried apricots — all shrink-wrapped in "health-food" packaging.

Enough fat to give a four-legged pig cardiac arrest.

To help Nance get to sleep after indulging myself with sweets, I pressed her temples and squeezed the back of her skull. She labeled my efforts "a great comfort."

Her words reminded me what touch can do. But it again exposed one of my partner's psychic holes: She'd grown up without intimacy. Her dad kept his proper Bostonian distance, from wife and daughter. Her mom believed affection was 110 percent private, that even public hugging was an embarrassment — and that feelings should be avoided and not discussed. Hardly the galaxy's best role models.

I'd been teaching her to fight for closeness; she's been learning.

Slowly.

Friday, Feb. 10

The chemo has knocked Nancy flatter than a fallen soufflé. Three pre-scheduled visitors watched her sleep today.

Saturday, Feb. 11

Nancy was wiped out for the second day in a row. She slept almost around the clock.

The cumulative effect of the chemo has been savage, arduous to witness.

In spite of her fatigue, my wife joined me on a trip to the hardware store for a new doorbell. Her riding shotgun wasn't necessary but changing out of a robe into street clothes acted as an anti-depressant.

Sunday, Feb. 12

If a caregiver isn't paying close attention, the job can turn into a full-time gig.

It can mean, for example, being a one-man pet-sitter, nurse, servant and counselor (all in the same time period). Today it meant I had to feed our dog and cat, brew tea when my wife got thirsty, raise the heat when she felt cold and turn it off when she felt warm, straighten covers she continually threw off and on, shop for Fuji apples because they're her favorite, install a new doorbell so she could hear visitors from the bedroom downstairs, listen to her daughter during a brief visit tell us she had to rush back to her place to prepare for a tomorrow flight to L.A., and hear my spouse repeat again and again that she has "the energy of a slug."

Whew!

On my short trip to "the outer world," an AM station played tunes hooked into Tuesday's holiday. "My Funny Valentine" — our song — was featured. My eyes misted.

I'm fragile, persistently on the verge of tears. Part of my sadness, which can dangle like an overweight albatross, has devolved in part from Nancy's barrage of identical questions. Those queries, to trace the horror backward, were caused by the chemo that damaged her short-term memory.

"I'm cold," she repeated tonight. "Why am I cold? Was it like this the other times — first cold, then hot, then cold?"

Were that not difficult enough, her insecurities have run wild. Woody: "Do you want more tea?" Nance: "No, I want you to hold me. I want you to get into bed and hold me. Hold me."

Monday, Feb. 13

During her group today, Nancy recognized she's among those who've "already been through the stuff the new patients are experiencing." The insight caused a momentary up.

Tuesday, Feb. 14

Stupid mistake! I asked Nancy to list her post-cancer symptoms so I'd be aware of all she's been through. Putting them on paper became a full-bodied bummer. For both of us.

What she listed, in no order of importance or irritation, were: "Rash from drug allergy, headaches, fatigue, nausea, common cold, shortness of breath, cough, sciatica, yeast infection, sores in mouth, sleeplessness, infection where drain from operation broke skin, soreness in shoulder and arm and back from lymph operation, hair loss, inability to concentrate, loss of memory, loss of appetite, metallic taste in mouth, light-headedness from smells, diarrhea, sore throat."

And she didn't list two that seem constant — an inability to grip anything firmly, so she keeps dropping things, and "chemo-brain," a catchall phrase covering a gamut of memory and cognitive lapses that would be validated by a Stanford University study released in November 2011.

All in all, just enough to make her a teensy-weensy crabby.

And she didn't even have to deal with the horrific menopausal symptoms a lot of middle-aged women with breast cancer must endure at the same time they're undergoing treatments.

Wednesday, Feb. 15

Nancy received top healing grades from her surgeon when she greeted him with both arms stretched way above her head, a feat she couldn't accomplish for a long time after what I keep calling a lymphectomy but what's more properly known in medical circles as an axillary lymph node dissection.

Thursday, Feb. 16

My wife discovered some of her jewelry has been stolen. At first she panicked. "Breathe," I said. "Breathe. In the big picture, it's not important."

After listing what was missing, she stared blankly through the kitchen window at a fat oak tree for a long time.

Finally, she admitted I was right. "What I feel in my heart is that I'm okay. You're okay. Nobody was threatened or shot. And the jewelry, though valuable in dollars, is not valuable when you measure it against life."

The burglary, peculiar because there was no sign of forced entry, "made me realize each day is vital and that doing what we want shouldn't be put off," she added. "I really want to fix our home, to travel, to enjoy our friends and recreation. I look forward to feeling well enough to get out more. Perhaps after Chemo No. 4. I hope, I hope."

Friday, Feb. 17

Nancy did some P.R. work at home, then walked with a friend for an hour and half. Her rule for the hike: "We will not talk about cancer." Our dog, who accompanied them, "insisted on dunking in every stream, and had a great time," my wife told me later. "It's so beautiful where we live."

Not so beautiful are the piles of chemicals my wife must ingest.

Her meds, not counting the ever-toxic chemo, include Prozac, to counteract depression, and a laundry list of stuff prescribed by her herbalist-acupuncturist.

She follows the holistic wizard's recommendations of Vitamins C and E and Selenium and Betacaratene, anti-oxidants all, to "seek out oxidized molecules that cause problems and also strengthen the immune system." And Gla 125 and Omega 3 Fatty Acids (flax seed oil), which are "of anti-inflammatory value." COQ10, which "promotes increased oxygen in the blood [and] circulation in the small capillaries," supposedly is a proven anti-cancer agent. Rei-Shi Gen, a peptide, also has reputed pro-immune value. And let's not ignore Siberian ginseng, which reputedly promotes white blood cell regeneration, or Thymus and Astrazalus, still more pro-immune substances.

It may be gobbledygook to me but the combo might be working. Nance seems to be faring better than most breast cancer patients at this point. Then, again, maybe it's just the "blood-cleansing teas" she's been guzzling.

Saturday, Feb. 18

Nancy's missing jewelry turned up — in a place she'd stashed it for protection. "As soon as I opened the drawer where they were hidden," she said sheepishly, "I remembered."

Later in the day we traveled to the home of a couple of friends, for dinner and laughter.

Both were copious, the latter primed by our playing Scrabble with the regulation that all words had to be invented and funny.

Tuesday, Feb. 21

Our lives seem dependent these days on what playwright Tennessee Williams called "the kindness of strangers," not an easy path for control freaks such as the two of us.

My fattened body is a head-to-toe portrait of my out-of-controlness, the result of emotional-hunger pleas for pound after pound of food. My mind, at the same time, struggles to learn how to hold things together with chewing gum and spit and two-sided tape — how to pretend the chaos isn't chaotic.

On the upside, our social worker extracted a promise that we'll touch each other when feeling alienated.

Wednesday, Feb. 22

My wife spent most of her psychotherapy session in anguish, talking about her daughter, "whose presence and devotion has been notably absent."

To pacify Nancy, I brought her a package of seedless red grapes (her favorite fruit), chocolate chip cookies (her junk-food preference) and frozen peanut-butter yogurt (her pseudo-health-food choice).

She grunted a thank-you but was in no rush to gobble down the stuff. Her lethargy dismayed me.

Thursday, Feb. 23

My wife ranked this evening's bodywork a total success. "Professional massages are among the highlights of my life right now," she noted.

Sunday, Feb. 26

A film we screened feels like the 1,739th mediocre video since Nance's diagnosis.

Monday, Feb. 27

Nancy and I spent most of our counseling hour writing down what's been good in our relationship. If I could sustain that perspective, I'd be as ecstatic as a retriever with a tennis ball in his cheek.

Thursday, March 2

Today warrants a checkmark on the calendar. Chemo treatment No. 4, the final ordeal, ended with a "graduation ceremony."

Nancy was given balloons, a "certificate of achievement" with her name imprinted, and hugs from all three nurses. Laughter blended with relief and good wishes.

The women in white also made sure to tell me I was a rarity. "Few men attend every session like you did," one of them noted.

Nance's inevitable fatigue didn't show up until after dinner. It arrived just as I handed her a small ceramic fox for her cluttered shelf of namesakes. "This animal is complete, intact," I said with unadulterated earnestness. "You are the same."

As she fondled the tiny sculpture, my wife accidentally snapped off a spindly rear leg. "Oh, God, throw it out," I said, my voice cracking. "It no longer represents who you are."

A second, more rational thought led me to phone the storekeeper to see if she had another. No such luck. But we could order one, which I did.

Because Nance can read me like an ABC primer, she could tell how shook up I was. I never admitted it, though. My silence went hand-in-glove with my hiding my darker thoughts more and more each week.

Wednesday, March 8

Today dashed by as Nancy and I composed a song for her mom. "That was great," said my partner. "Sometimes I forget how much fun we have working on creative projects."

My morning group had also been upbeat. A new guy said his wife's jaw had locked in an apparent allergic reaction to anti-nausea pills. The men joked about it, probably because it existed safely in the past tense. One participant noted it was a shame we couldn't bottle it. "Many a guy — not me, of course — would pay a small fortune to bolt his wife's jaw," he said.

Monday, March 13

Chuckles prevailed today in Nancy's support group, their origin being a tape satirizing guided visualizations.

Afterward, my wife went to her oncologist's office for a blood count. It was low again, so she had to swallow antibiotics for a third time. The cycle — chemo, fatigue, recovery; chemo, fatigue, recovery — has been consistent. But being predictable hasn't made it any easier to confront.

Nance's bravery continued to amaze me; it's been like a steady lighthouse beacon to a seaman in a hurricane. It's strengthened my strength.

Friday, March 17

The surgeon checked the site of Nancy's incision again. "It's discolored but healing appropriately," he advised in doctor-speak. "And your arm movement is first-rate."

Nance pointed to the underside. "There's no feeling at all," she said.

The doctor said she'll have to deal with her arm the rest of her life. She's not to lift anything over 15 pounds with it. She must avoid puncturing it in any way. Forever.

Because many of my wife's lymph nodes were removed, a permanent swelling from retention of water has become a permanent threat.

Wednesday, March 22

Nancy's psychiatrist apparently watched her sprint up and down an emotional escalator.

My wife told me they covered "priorities, how I feel about myself, what gives me pleasure, and how I feel about death, something I haven't articulated or explored with him."

The meaning of life has yet to emerge from the disease or its wake but what has become evident to both Nance and me is what is not important. The five hundred dollars it cost to fix my Toyota smelled like a rip-off but we wanted to move on with our lives. We had the car repaired without blinking.

"There's only one thing that's important — keeping well," said Nance. "The rest seems foolish."

Friday, March 24

Early today, in my shrink's office, I owned my indignation at Nancy's oncologist for having suggested another long-range treatment, a course of tamoxifen. I'd previously convinced myself, as had my wife, that the major treatments would end with radiation. Now Western medicine wanted to keep my wife sick five more years.

Much of what I'd heard about tamoxifen had been negative. And in a 90-minute phone conversation last weekend, my ex-wife catalogued her problems with the drug. She'd put on more than seventy pounds while fighting *her* breast cancer. She'd also been suffering from several other typical side effects of the medication — headaches, vaginal dryness, hot flashes.

My mind was stuck on a single question: "Is living a few extra months worth a giant erosion in quality of life?"

One statistic Nance's oncologist gave us led to our decision. Tamoxifen is effective in only ten percent of cases like my wife's, "where the cancer cells have negative hormone receptors."

Nance and I came up with the same answer: "Fergeddaboudit."

Monday, March 27

We went to an Academy Award costume party this evening. Nancy and I dressed as "Pulp Fiction" twins, each carrying oranges to suggest the pulp and wearing pinned-on pages from the National Enquirer to symbolize the fiction. To some degree, my wife found the party "refreshing, because many people didn't know I am battling cancer."

But a late appearance of her ex-lover caused a major bump in the night. We'd run into him many times before without a snag. Tonight, however, he came cloaked in black, as Death, his partner wearing bridal white (representing "Four Weddings and a Funeral").

Nance instantly became weirded out. Her reaction came on the heels of a bad dream last night. In it, she'd been given the choice of devouring our golden retriever or dying. She chose the latter.

"I don't feel safe," she'd said then, waking me seconds after she'd awakened. "Rub my back. Hold me."

Wednesday, March 29

I took the day off so I could accompany Nancy to the radiologist's office.

The doctor patiently answered each of our questions. Then she barred me from the radiation-room simulation.

While I brooded about being left out, Nance lay motionlessly on a table. As huge machines plucked from a science-fiction movie whirled around her body, the ceiling offered a painted view of a leafy sky that was supposed to pacify her. It didn't. The technicians worked swiftly, drawing X's and other marks on her breast, pinpointing where the radiation will strike. Two dot-sized tattoos became permanent decorations. My mate was grateful for the technology but detested having to be there.

Thursday, March 30

The radiologist had scheduled a cat-scan (also called a CT or, more precisely, "computed tomography") for Nancy at 7 a.m.

"It feels like millions of people have touched my breasts, moved them around, palpated them, made marks on them," my wife said later.

In the afternoon, she returned to the hospital for a mammogram, which she described as "an exercise in which I put my breasts on a cold steel shelf, one at a time, and a cold machine makes pancakes out of them, first horizontally, then vertically. To make the breasts fit right, a techie with cold hands pulls and tugs at them as if they were Silly Putty.

"Can you imagine what it would feel like if they did that to your penis?"

Nance's third experience at the hospital today turned out to be the worst.

We'd been scheduled for an evening counseling session with our social worker, whose office is in the same building as the oncologist's. But when the radiologist saw us in the waiting room, she asked if we'd come in for a minute. She was stone-faced. That felt ominous.

In fact, they'd found a microscopic spot on the mammogram.

Prognosis: Probably another lumpectomy, regardless of whether it's cancer or a calcification of some kind. "Protective surgery." And another wait, this time for the surgeon to confirm and to set a date for the outpatient procedure.

The cause? "Perhaps the lumpectomy surgery itself, perhaps an undiscovered cancer," said the female radiologist. "No one's sure."

Nance and I both felt as if we'd fallen from the rollercoaster and been crushed under its wheels. The doctor hugged my partner, then me. Her warmth failed to erase my distress.

"I'm not happy," said Nance under the comparative safety of our roof. "I'm angry inside, though I didn't realize it in the radiologist's office. I'm sad I might have to go through still another surgical procedure. I'm sick of procedures. I'm sick of having knives and machines and hands and marking pens stuck in my body."

Saturday, April 1

We waited for the surgeon to call.

The day dragged and dragged and dragged. I drew a parallel to being in downtown San Francisco during the big earthquake of '89. I'd discovered quickly that the experts had lied about how to find a refuge. There was no safe place, nowhere to hide, nowhere to run. Slivers of glass and chunks of brick fell from skyscrapers. Streets arched. Electric wires sparked and died. Insecurity and shock invaded my every pore.

Insomnia had hounded me after the quake. Last night, riddled with cancer fears, was a repeat.

Sunday, April 2

The surgeon still didn't phone.

Nancy eventually ran out of distractions so she dialed his answering service. Her exasperation swelled. A second doctor was covering and her surgeon was beyond reach.

"Shit" was all she said.

Monday, April 3

The waiting has been driving me batty. I'm a semi-official pacifist but I've had a demented urge to break something or hit someone, to give me the feeling I have a smidgen of control.

My concentration has gone into slow motion, like a villain being pushed through a picture window in a classic Bruce Willis action movie.

Nancy's support group was empathetic with her impatience, but its members were impotent, too.

When at last she reached the surgeon mid-afternoon, his answer was infuriatingly indecisive. Although he was "pretty sure the spot isn't cancer," he suggested another mammogram. Since the lab can't schedule my partner until the day after tomorrow, it means more waiting. And, of course, even more after that for the results.

Shit!

Tuesday, April 4

Nance and I normally fought for the reins. Now we've been forced to let medical practitioners take over.

Neither of us has enjoyed that.

"I want to be in charge of my own body but can't," Nance admitted, her voice cracking.

In our entire marriage, the tension has never been this extreme. I've felt more and more alienated. I've been short-fused, then apologetic. Instead of wanting to be a caregiver, I've wished to curl into a fetal ball and let out a bloodcurdling scream. I've often wept behind closed doors, or been on the verge of crying.

I'd like someone to deliver about five tons of armor plate to shield my mind and heart.

Wednesday, April 5

A radiologist-friend became our guardian angel again by agreeing to read the latest mammogram quickly.

After consulting with his colleagues, and within two hours of the procedure, he told our message machine the trouble spot was "round, with no soft tissue, and not suspicious."

Deciphered into English, it's not another cancer and there's no need for surgery.

Nance, who'd mentally prepared herself for a second lumpectomy, was elated. Me, too.

Thursday, April 6

My wife scooted to the hospital for a radiation run-through. "It was fast, scientific, computer-driven, efficient," she said. "The actual therapy will be a breeze. The side effects — well, they're still to be determined."

6

THE WAY MEN SEE IT

I sometimes equate Marin Man to Man with a vitamin supplement.

Our weekly support group — or any other like it anywhere else — can keep guys feeling healthy, or give them a crucial boost when the walls of their lives seem to be caving in.

Actually, because of its collective experience, the group can be a supplement in multiple ways:

We can complement Internet info, factoids and data, often differentiating between truth and fiction. We can de-code what physicians and other healers say — and don't say. We can increase the understanding offered by relatives, friends and co-workers because we frequently empathize when they can't. We can — without embarrassment — be warm and friendly, direct and anecdotal, and add an intimacy factor because we're human beings and not a book, journal, chat-room or blog. We can increase a newbie's stockpile of contacts and where-do-you-find-its because we've been there.

Best of all, we can be ultra-illuminating because we can share what's worked for us and what hasn't.

For two decades Man to Man has attracted fellows habitually willing to be candid about themselves and their partners, about their day-terrors and exhausting triumphs, about their feet of clay and feats of unsung heroism while facing a breast cancer rollercoaster.

They're unusual: They show up. They listen. They talk.

The vast majority of men are unwilling to be that open. They're too afraid to display their fear.

They're afraid to be vulnerable.

John Teasley is a guy who overcame a Texas brainwashing that insisted he "ask no personal questions nor show any emotions."

But after his wife underwent a double mastectomy, reconstructive surgery and chemo, he recognized he "needed help coping" — not with just his wife's survival but his.

So he swallowed his pride and came to his first Man to Man breakfast. Years later, he still attends.

At Marin-Man-to-Man.org he notes that it "has provided a sounding board for sensitive health issues and made me realize that I was not alone in my ordeal or fears."

Marv Edelstein writes — on the same site — that the group still provides him "an outlet for fears that surface every time [my wife] experiences a strange pain or ailment, or a friend experiences a recurrence."

He admits that when he first heard about Man to Man his "immediate reaction was stereotypically male: "Support group? I don't need one."

Ultimately he couldn't "come up with a legitimate reason to say no," so he agreed to join in.

He's been ordering the breakfast-and-conversation special each week for 20 years, finding his initial hesitation "to be completely unwarranted… This was a place to ask questions, get answers to questions I hadn't thought to ask, and find comfort in the realization that what I was experiencing was no different than what everyone else was going through."

Dan Goltz remembers the breast cancer and subsequent treatments hitting "like a tornado, whirling us into a terrible depression. [My wife] suffered the pain and discomfort, but I felt the ever-present fear that my wonderful wife could die. It was devastating."

He also recalls showing up at a weekly Man to Man meeting "full of apprehension about meeting new people I assumed would be as miserable as I was. But it wasn't that way at all, [and] to my surprise, I was able to talk freely about how I felt. The other men listened, asked questions and gave me advice [as well as] my first gleam of hope that maybe things could turn out okay."

Things did.

As a bonus, he ended up making "wonderful lasting friendships" in the group.

That was particularly helpful when, years later, his wife "had a second bout — not a recurrence but a whole new strain. I'm a big baseball fan so it was natural for me to think, 'Wow, this is like playing a doubleheader. But we were able to win the first one, so we should be able to win this one, too.' And we did."

Not every guy escapes his breast cancer trials unscathed.

John Sundberg got loads of help as a Man to Man regular. But his wife died.

His initial visit, just prior to her beginning treatments, was hard. He wanted to know what chemo "was really like, [and] what I heard scared me so much I could hardly breathe, much less eat my breakfast.

"They told me what I needed to hear, what no one else could. I really appreciated their honesty. I need to stop living the 'it's not happening to me' world and face the reality of chemotherapy and breast cancer, so that I could be there to support my wife."

On our website, he observes that, while the "group had good ideas about medical treatments and opinions about local doctors and hospitals," he found that "best of all, I could just be myself...I could be discouraged, frustrated or angry, and it was okay."

When breast cancer finally claimed his wife, members of the support group participated in the memorial service.

He kept going to the sessions for several years afterward.

Gerry Borguignon also became a regular, but not because of his wife. He contracted breast cancer himself.

Requiring a modified mastectomy.

And then a course of tamoxifen, stopping it after 18 months because of "increasingly painful side effects" that "apparently...are generally worse for men compared to women."

He joined Man to Man after feeling "rather 'alone' regarding how to deal with my situation as a cancer survivor."

Online, he offers one more variation on a heavily repetitive theme: Men need support despite their fondness of believing they can "fix it" themselves — the "it" being almost anything.

Paul Thompson described himself in an early version of our site as having once been a guy "most comfortable being independent; being able to solve my own problems; never feeling the need to build a circle of male friends to just 'pal around with.'"

But when his wife's breast cancer diagnosis was handed down, he knew he "needed help in working through the maze of choices and uncertainties associated with the disease. Furthermore, I knew that the help I needed was not the clinical kind that one gets from the oncologist or psychiatrist, but the down-to earth, 'I've been there' help that can only come from another man who has experienced what I'm experiencing."

He got that from the men — over and over.

While no groups parallel to Marin Man to Man exist in the San

Francisco Bay Area, some do function in other states. In fact, when Paul Thompson and his wife relocated to Eugene, Oregon, he started "a look-alike group" there.

Ours, meanwhile, is likely to meet for many more years, with our members continuing to range from those whose partners have had a lumpectomy, a single mastectomy or a double to the rare guys who've contracted breast cancer themselves.

Future regulars or occasional drop-ins, as in the past, are likely to include professionals, tradesmen, the unemployed, from every socioeconomic level, of every age, faith and skin color.

It is unlikely, though, that we'll draw even one dude stuck on being "Macho Man."

7
RADIATION

I'd edited special-edition newspapers immediately after the assassination of John F. Kennedy and the San Francisco earthquake of 1989, and would do so again the day terrorists took down the World Trade Center in New York. Each time I had difficulty keeping my feelings at arm's length. But I did, at least until the papers were being delivered. Only then did I give myself permission to cry.

Throughout Nancy's treatments, I'd put out a series of regular papers. I never learned to de-personalize the breast cancer, though. And while I'd displayed few of my feelings to co-workers during the weeks of radiation, the dizzying sensations had continually bombarded me — as ubiquitously as TV commercials.

Friday, April 7

Today, the first of 33 radiation days, gorged us with emotion.

My stomach became a volcano as I stared at Nancy. She lay on her back, motionless, filling the narrow, padded hospital platform. Her right arm was raised in an artificial stirrup salute to the hallowed god of techno-medicine. Red rays peeked through holes in the ceiling, and lined up with a magic-marker blueprint on her bare right breast.

In spite of the techies and doc doing everything imaginable to comfort us, in spite of orderlies having antiseptically scrubbed the place so everything shined, eeriness polluted the pre-conditioned air.

As if trapped in a bad horror flick, I fully expected a hunchbacked lackey named Igor to lunge from a dank passageway.

I had no idea how Nance was reacting but I grew more uncomfortable with each passing second. My father had coached me when I was a toddler: "Nuclear energy and radiation are evil, to be avoided and fought at all costs; neither belong in the fallible hands of man."

Because brainwashing dies hard, it became difficult for me to accept the possibility radiation could save Nance's life instead of kill her.

Images of Hiroshima and Ten-Mile Island played hide-and-seek inside my head. Nance's face morphed from the mushroom clouds and meltdown sites.

To soothe herself, my wife activated an internal anesthetic device. She was convinced that becoming wooly-brained was her best way to cope because she was totally vulnerable, at the mercy of the nuts and bolts.

"What I did," she explained, "was kill any feelings whatsoever that popped up by focusing on visualizations."

Earlier in the day, an expert in guided imagery had led her through one at the hospital.

"I saw a small figure in a canoe in the ocean," Nance told her. "The waves were huge but the person kept paddling and was not swept under.

"Then I remembered the watercolor hanging near our front door. It depicts a woman resting on turbulent waters — with a cat peacefully sleeping on her chest. It's always represented the ability to be peaceful in the midst of chaos."

During the meditative exercise, Nance said, "I entered the picture and became that woman. I suddenly became aware God was crying above me. Tears filled the sky but as they fell they were transformed into webs that descended toward me in straight, strong lines, like beautiful spider silk. The webs attached to me and kept me afloat, providing me with strength."

The visualization guide then asked if there were any other issues she wanted to confront. "Yes," said my wife. "I want to protect my skin during radiation."

"How will you do that?"

Without faltering, Nance described wrapping the breast "with the same materials spun from the tears of God. It protects my skin but allows the healing rays to penetrate the cancer site."

Saturday, April 8

Counting our blessings was a cinch today. Two friends helped us fill our time with laughter, companionship, hearty walks, excellent food and a trio of W's — wildflowers, water and whales.

"This is the kind of day I love," commented Nancy, "a day that makes me glad to be alive."

Scattered showers failed to erase our pleasure. We simply picnicked in the car, in an information-station parking lot on the way to the shore, and watched raindrops dribble down the windows.

The last dark cloud sailed into the distance just as we crumpled our paper napkins.

Minutes later, from the base of a lighthouse, we spied a huge gray whale.

A scrumptious dinner at a nearby inn topped it all off.

For me, it was a day of renewal. I'd nearly forgotten how fantastic it can be to spend time in the fresh air, how I relax when near the ocean or bay.

It's oneness. It's fun.

It's life affirming.

Sunday, April 9

Cancer can't be wholly blamed for Nancy's short-term memory loss; she's suffered from a touch of it for years. But chemo has intensified the problem. Lately, she's disremembered things from one sentence to the next. And the gaps in her recall scare her so much she fumes when she notices that I notice.

But a major lesson for us has been to accept and — as advocates in scores of disciplines believe — let God run the show.

While we were working toward that ethereal status, Nance pressed her fight to retain control. She scribbled self-reminders as fast as a five-dollar caricaturist whipped out drawings. And like weeds in front of a home in foreclosure, the yellow stickies multiplied exponentially. They not only covered the refrigerator but the staircase railing, the bathroom medicine cabinet, the front door.

"I have lists and notes all over the place, and I do the things I write down. The rest go unremembered, undone."

My thought when she said that: *"Maybe that's life's bottom line — unfinished business."*

Monday, April 10

Following her second hit of radiation, Nance met with her doctor and complained about a rib hurting. The radiologist said she'd check the x-ray from a couple of months ago and, if need be, order another film.

I, at work, thought every third second about what my partner was going through. She'd thanked me profusely for being at each of her chemo sessions and her first radiation gig, then reassured me — after consulting with the radiologist — she could do the rest of the series alone.

It didn't matter who'd given her an okay, however. I accumulated guilt from not being there for each nuking.

Saturday, April 15

Saturdays have begun to annoy me from top to bottom. They've become chock full of trivial tasks that preclude anything substantial.

Today we added several hours of car shopping to our usual mix. We admitted being excited about the possibility of buying one, but making a decision may be difficult: Our heads aren't screwed on straight, and haven't been for months.

Want the consummate example of our being discombobulated? After Nancy plopped down for a two-hour rest, we rushed to a nearby theater for a young songwriters' concert. We arrived minutes before curtain time — a full week early.

Too weary to be humiliated, we laughed. "Let's go to a movie," I suggested.

The mediocre substitution — the latest example of our new motif of living in the here-and-now — showed us we'd prefer nearly anything to returning home and thinking about breast cancer.

Sunday, April 16

Nancy dreamed about kissing my ear and arousing me. Upon awakening, she pulled me back into bed to make it happen. We cradled each other after the sex, peaceful and happy.

"I love being close and warm," she said, "and love forgetting for the moment that I'm a patient and I'm bald."

Speaking of hairlessness, a little stubble had pierced Nance's chin, the last place on her body she wanted fuzz. Nevertheless, it became an omen of recovery, making us both smile. "By the hair of your chinny-chin-chin," I sang gleefully, "it's a sure sign you're getting better and gonna beat this thing."

Monday, April 17

In the middle of the night, Nancy awoke with a severe headache. She urged me to press into her skull, a mission she's suggested repeatedly since the chemo began. The pressure from my fingers apparently relieves the pain. I sometimes ache from the strain but don't stop because her suffering is greater.

Tuesday, April 18

Nancy sprinted through public relations odds and ends at home after this morning's radiation, then met a friend for lunch. According to my wife, they "talked about our lives, our families, our hopes, our health" — apparently leaving out only rocket science and the merits of a flat-tax.

For the time being, however, her priority can't be conversation. Rather, it must be on keeping her irradiated breast as trouble-free as possible. To increase her chances, she's been rubbing on Ching Wan Hong, an alternative burn cream, along with Theracare, the ointment her radiologist pushed.

A little East, a little West.

Thankfully, there's been only a slight discoloration so far, and no burning.

Wednesday, April 19

Stress has disfigured Nance's face. The effects of surgery, chemo and radiation have made her look older, pale, haggard. More importantly, she's plagued by a devastating listlessness that requires napping a couple of hours, day after day. On the rare occasions when I go out at night, she's typically asleep when I arrive home. When I awaken for work, she's usually snoring. Sometimes I don't see her hazel eyes all day, and can talk on the phone for only a minute or two.

Not quite conducive to intimacy.

My soulmate's new F-words, fatigue and forgetfulness, have been — like labor pains — coming closer and closer together. "I'm really tired," she said with a wan smile tonight. "And I'm really tired of being sick."

Worrying about her has further truncated my own sleep-time. The bags under my eyes look like squooshed pink jelly beans.

Thursday, April 20

Radiation No. 10.

The treatment has become the first nail with which Nancy cobbles together each morning — "certainly an odd way for a person to start the day," she noted.

Oddly warm, too.

"The people waiting for treatments are friendly," she noted. "We all encourage each other. The more personal details we learn, the more comfortable we get. It may sound strange to call it that, but it's a little community."

Sunday, April 23

Nancy and I verbally revisited the mellow chat we'd had the other day on a bank of the creek here in San Anselmo. We agreed it resurrected our tenderness.

That pleasant feeling was reinforced as we planned a brief European vacation to follow the treatments.

And the sensation got an extra boost when two friends came over for a "catered Chinese dinner" in the usual little white cardboard cartons. Foursome fun. What's always most terrific about the twosome is their authenticity, unpretentiousness and honesty. Rare qualities in a cynical world.

The day's *piéce de résistance*, so to speak, was truly good sex. "I've had 47 orgasms," proclaimed my wife with an enormous grin, exaggerating by at least 44.

Even with such barefaced overstatement, the female capacity for multiple climaxes once again leaves me envious.

Monday, April 24

"I look like a freshly-shaved beard, but my hair's growing back and it's soft," exclaimed Nancy with no mean degree of wonderment and joy. "I don't know what color it is, but it's dark with white patches. I can't wait till I have real hair."

She also discovered stubble on her legs, chin and pubic mound.

As a result, she glowed like a tot covered with sparkling fingerpaint. The irony was that a portion of her radiance came from acquiring hair on her legs, where she's more than once wished she had no growth at all.

Wednesday, April 26

This evening, when I told Nancy I wanted to crash without dinner, she said I couldn't. "Why not?" I asked with a tone that could curdle milk.

"Because I've planned a surprise," she said.

As we neared dinner's end, she piped up: "The massage person will be here in a few minutes. You should get into a robe."

My twinkle couldn't have been brighter.

"Timing is everything," a wise man once said — or was that a watchmaker? Although Nance usually enjoys massages more than I, tonight was an exception: The tightness in my shoulders resembled a swollen steel bar.

The masseuse firmly yet tenderly kneaded my muscles, first buffing my torso with oils to help soften my skin, relieve my tension and make her work easier.

I was asleep on the portable massage table within five minutes.

An hour later, I not only shone from oil but from love. It awed me that Nance could reach beyond her pains and anxieties to please me with the gift of relaxation.

Friday, April 28

Attitude about breast cancer — or anything else, probably — is a crucial element any day of the week.

My bus, in the midst of a huge traffic jam, was trapped between stops today. A nattily accessorized African American with a skinny leather briefcase paced uncomfortably. Every three or four seconds, he'd check his watch.

Finally, exasperated, he shouted at the driver, also African American. "Lemme off! Now!"

Quietly, the driver said, "I can't. It's dangerous, and if you were to be injured, the city would be liable."

"Fuck you," snarled the passenger, hoisting his briefcase over his head. "I'm late, and I'm getting later every minute. Lemme off or I'll slam you with this."

"Do what you gotta do," said the driver with unbelievable calm.

In response, the antagonist slammed his briefcase into the double-fold front door. The panes cracked, fashioning a modern-art piece. But no glass fell.

Again and again the man futilely pounded at the doors with his fists.

The handful of seated passengers, myself included, tried to shrink into as tiny and invisible a space as possible. No one knew what this maniac would do next.

"Lemme out," he screamed again at the driver. "Lemme out, nigger."

"Do what you gotta do," repeated the driver. "I gotta follow orders." Not a single bead of perspiration dotted his forehead.

The traffic jam suddenly dissolved, and the bus was able to ease forward to the next stop. The driver opened the doors as if nothing beyond the ordinary had happened. The glass-breaker vaulted out, disappearing in a run down a side street.

"My God," a woman said to the busman, "how'd you stay so calm?"

Replied the driver, "I'm a Buddhist and when he started to shout I started a mental mantra that brings me peace. I let go of the problem."

Saturday, April 29

I kept thinking today how blessed we are. Ten years ago — maybe even less — Nancy's treatment would have consisted of lopping off her breast.

Period. No options. No questions asked.

I'm thrilled, too, about Nance's hair growing back, soft and smooth — it means so much to her. But she's been driving me nuts asking, "What color is it? Can you tell what color it is?"

Wednesday, May 3

Nancy pretended her head was a debutante today: She gave it a coming-out party.

After her 8 a.m. radiation, she took a long walk, winding up at a cafe in the next town. She was sweaty and her scalp was hot. She pondered why she kept her hat on when all she wanted was to remove it. Off it went.

"To my amazement, there was no audible gasp in the restaurant," she said. "The diners didn't stand en masse and point at my head. No hair-police ticketed me. All that happened was that I was comfortable. It was a victorious moment."

Friday, May 5

Nancy has been treating a newly developed rash on her chest with a steroid cream. "It itches like hell," she wailed artificially, her theatrical way of begging for sympathy.

One breath later she said, "This should be the worst thing that happens to me. Miracle of miracles, I am not burned. Only 12 more times. Only 12 more."

She's been so convinced she's healing she's had zero objections to my taking a business trip to Finland, Russia and Sweden.

By all rights I should have been ecstatic. I haven't been. Although it'll be good to escape the tensions of the newspaper and the anxiety of the radiation, although there are countless friends and acquaintances and medical personnel around to help her, I've felt guilty about the chance Nance will burn and I won't be here for comfort.

Sunday, May 7

The highlight of Nancy's day, while I was jetting across the Atlantic toward Helsinki, was going to "Angels in America, Part I" with a computer-artist friend.

Before leaving for the theater in San Francisco, she'd shown my partner a bunch of images she'd stylized. They depicted the changes Nance had endured. My wife selected half a dozen shots to reproduce on a thank-you letter for those who've supported her.

Her favorite?

One in which a bouquet of flowers sprouted from her pate.

Monday, May 8

Today, Nancy would tell me much later, was tainted by a classic medical horror.

The incident was exactly what I'd dreaded — something bad happening and my not being present to support her.

After radiation treatment No. 22, the technicians had asked Nance to simulate being zapped by a new machine that would send a radiation boost precisely to the vicinity where her cancer originated.

"My head was placed in a molded plastic form so I couldn't move it in either direction," she reported. "As I lay there, the technician moved the machine too close to my chin, forcing my head to turn while the plastic held me tight. I felt like my neck was going to snap."

It was an accident, they said — "human error."

Nance's radiologist said it "had never happened before" but, as a result, they were "going to change the procedure." She expressed compassion, but the damage had been done.

Nance cried throughout the simulation. "The tears just kept coming," she said. "I felt so small, so helpless. I knew how much power the machine had over me at that moment, and how much trust I've placed in doctors and technicians who are subject to 'human error.' I don't like being the human on whom they are erring."

She also wept, she said, "because the cancer, like the machine, is very big. Very big. And like the machine, I can exert no control over it except what I do with my mind, which is why I've been working so hard to stay focused and positive."

Her summary: "I feel so vulnerable. I didn't need this. At all."

Nance's support group chanced to be meeting shortly thereafter, so she provided "the girls" details of what had happened.

She found receptive ears.

The meeting became a major downer, though, because the next to talk was a member who'd just had a recurrence, the sword of Damocles that hangs over every breast cancer patient's head.

The woman first experienced breast cancer eight years ago. She told of dealing with the idea of death, about how she's been focused about staying in the moment but worried she won't see her 12-year-old daughter grow up.

Several participants used the news to say they'd become more spiritual during the cancer experience. Others reported plans for vacations, unwilling to wait until next year or retirement or more disease.

Saturday, May 13

Nancy joined her friend to see "Perestroika," the second part of the play "Angels in America." And she called me in Stockholm.

I wasn't in my room so she left a message. Then she wrote in her diary, "It's been quiet, peaceful and restful while Woody's been away, but I miss him and love him and want him by my side to share my life."

As the evening progressed, her anxieties grew as high as a tsunami — the life-and-death themes of the play seemed to kick them into top gear.

She phoned again, waking me in the middle of a night that had been filled with rain and snow flurries. Most of the call we alternated saying "I love you."

She said zilch about her neck injury, about it being stiff and sore, or about her needing repeated massages.

Tuesday, May 16

Radiation No. 27 yesterday was followed by Nancy's support-group session and a trip to the Napa Valley wine country for an overnighter with a friend before a hot-air balloon ride early today.

Nance has wanted to do that forever. My inner-ear imbalance precluded my joining her. So my absence made this the perfect time. She described the experience — and her taking an extra day's respite from the radiation — as fantastic. "It was simply gorgeous floating up there."

Wednesday, May 17

After lunch, Nancy and another friend made plans to bake cupcake breasts when the radiation ordeal ends. They picked up some flesh-colored tint for the icing, and muffin tins shaped like boobs. "I'll give 'em to the doctors, therapists, librarians and chemotherapy nurses who've helped me," Nance said.

The massage person, shortly thereafter, gave her a two-hour neck rubdown, courtesy of a radiation department apparently trying to ward off a potential malpractice suit.

Thursday, May 18

Nancy may be more forgiving than I might have been.

Today was nuclear zapping No. 29. Only four more. Right after the treatment, Nance led the technician to a quiet place and said she pardoned him for his simulation screw-up. He seemed relieved.

Friday, May 19

The computer artist delivered the thank-you cards mid-afternoon. Nancy was pleased with the overall product and its message. The final version included six distorted, abstract photos of her during this time of crisis and regrowth.

To me, it was a joy she had the balls to be bald photographically.

In the evening, Nance met three women from her group and drove into San Francisco for dinner and a lecture by breast cancer doctor-expert Susan Love.

One point had particular impact.

Love recommended women in my wife's circumstances not take tamoxifen unless they were part of a study group. Her opinion solidified Nance's decision to skip the drug.

Love blamed a lot on environment and early use of radiation in the '40s, '50s and '60s.

But mostly, she said, cancer's a mystery.

Saturday, May 20

Nancy picked me up at the airport, gushed that she "couldn't wait to see me" and that she was happy I was safely on the ground. It's fascinating how virtually no one in the world is fully comfortable about those big metal birds that keep buzzing around the globe.

Sunday, May 21

Nancy wanted to hear every detail of my non-adventures but I delayed relating them until she filled me in about her health. When she brought me up to speed, I became outraged about the neck incident.

Monday, May 22

We tried sex again. It didn't work — again. We couldn't overcome Nancy's vaginal soreness. Chemo and cancer have been co-villains.

Tuesday, May 23

No. 32, the penultimate radiation treatment.

Following the therapy, Nancy's friend arrived with all the necessary groceries, accessories and equipment for baking six dozen cupcakes. The two co-conspirators dyed the sour cream cake-mix flesh color, then topped it with a Grand Marnier frosting. To create an areola look, they layered a darker hue.

The final touch, bubble-gum-colored jelly-bean nipples.

They baked and frosted, baked and frosted, most of the time singing and dancing. Shortly after they began, they stripped to the waist. That, according to my wife, "was a spontaneous and appropriate act since we were hot in the kitchen, and the whole thing was about breasts anyway."

Wednesday, May 24

Today's last radiation treatment brought nothing but happiness.

For Nancy, the day's secondary highlight became the distribution of her cupcakes. But she and I also celebrated with her daughter at a mountaintop inn. The food and wine were forgettable, the memory everlasting — because Nance's daughter presented her with two dozen white roses.

Just before going to bed, my wife wrote in her journal:

"Woody's return, the end of my treatments, the celebration about these endings — they were all highs for me. I also recognize God has helped me, that I am blessed, that I am lucky, that I am cured.

"This six months of treatment has been a rollercoaster that travels up, down, sideways, backwards, and in twists and turns, but always moves toward its final destination. I remember much of it very well. Other parts fade. I remember the emotions, the shock, the sadness, the determination, the hope, the annoyance, the pain. Mostly I remember putting one foot in front of another and keeping on.

"I remember Woody's fine advice on how to organize, prioritize, trivia-exorcise. I have learned how to let the minutiae go. I have learned to rest, to stop. I have learned to share more with Woody. I have learned a level of honesty with myself that I never dared have before.

"I have discussed with Woody what I would I do if I had three months to live, or six months, or 20 months. Or 20 years.

"I have considered what I want in my life. Peace, love, harmony, an end to war throughout the world. Those desires have not changed. But now I want to pay more attention to Woody, be a better mother and daughter.

"I have allowed myself to befriend visualizations, crystals, vitamins, hands-on healing. I have prayed.

"I want this entry in my diary to be profound. I want to remember all the important things, to put them down for me and Woody and whoever to see. But I don't feel profound. I simply feel relieved, so glad it's over.

"It was climbing through primordial slime; it was dealing with my dragons, my worst fears; it was embracing the unembraceable: my own sicknesses; it was loving a body that was alien to me, trusting that my real self would magically reappear. It was the knowledge that my real self is now different, a subtly colored butterfly with scars on its wings and short hairs on its head. But it is a butterfly, isn't it?"

8

AFTERMATH

Nancy's last radiation treatment shadowed the chemotherapy as closely as the paparazzi trail celebrities. On the first anniversary of her final nuclear session, I encouraged her to review where she'd been.

She wrote about her changed perspective:

"Because of the cancer, little things bug me a lot less. They frequently fall into the 'Oh, well' category. Oh, well, there's a stain on my favorite shirt. Oh, well, the critter peed on the rug.

"And the things that aren't 'oh, wells' are much clearer.

"Come to think of it, today is too precious to spend any more time at this keyboard. I'm hungry for a big taste of the day. I am a survivor."

I, too, had the constant feeling that I'd survived.

Because of those sensations, both of us believed we needed to give something back to the cancer community that facilitated our achieving that status.

So, a little less than half a year after Nancy's 33rd and final radiation treatment, we took part in a public discussion at Marin General Hospital on breast cancer. And we found ourselves surprised that one panelist, who'd climbed a real-life mountain after her diagnosis, assumed a posture of invincibility.

Only while stepping down from the platform did she confess, in private to us, that the illness had pushed her into a six-month funk.

A second panelist, a male public relations pro who'd self-published a pamphlet on being a caregiver, publicly offered a string of bumper-sticker slogans. His wife spoke glowingly of having been anesthetized for a mastectomy, then awakening with a smile and a reconstructed breast.

Nance and I stood out: We weren't 100 percent sanguine.

We told the audience of our having grown closer, but we also cited a gamut of emotions, strains on our marriage, and our alarm at learning we'd have to deal with cancer — even with the malignancy gone — the rest of our lives.

The program coordinator later praised us for not being "supermen or women, just yourselves, sometimes challenged, sometimes triumphant in the journey to wellness."

Our after-care journey also included putting our money and energy where our hope was.

Whenever the impulse hit us, we gave small sums for cancer studies. I donated my skills by redesigning a newsletter for a group that raised funds for breast cancer research. And my wife started contributing with her feet. The five-kilometer run/walk in Golden Gate Park raised hundreds of thousands of dollars annually and drew hordes of participants and watchers. Its $18 entry fee was perfect for those of us who embraced "chai," a Hebrew symbol representing both that numeral and the word "life."

It was essential, of course, for Nance to perceive her life was right side up again. So she worked at it.

"After I finished my treatments," she wrote, *"I immediately set about to prove to myself that I was a hundred percent. I resumed work, caring for my home and pets and plants, seeing friends, trying to do it all.*

"But I've learned to respect my middle-aging and the cancer toll on me and Woody by slowing down a bit."

Both of us found it impossible to climb immediately to previous fifth-gear levels, to the hectic life we'd considered normal. Nevertheless, we tried to cram as many diversions as possible into our "new normal" lifestyle.

"A lot's still not happening," wrote my wife. *"Having put aside almost everything for a full year, there's a backlog of home maintenance, projects we want to do, vacations we want to take, old friends we want to get together with. We try to do a little at a time but we both feel like we're always playing catch-up.*

"The banner headline, though, is: 'I am alive!' That stays with me always. I never thought about it before. I never thought, 'I am a living, breathing person on this Earth, and it feels fabulous just to be here.' I now think that thought very often."

Life-affirming precepts frequently eased our way — during and following the grueling year of treatments, and, I expect, they will do so forever.

Thinking about (and looking forward to) the annual Race for the Cure, for example, could always be counted on as a cheerer-upper. It pleased us to recognize that it and similar fund-raising events help underwrite research that, despite sky-high price tags, could become a wellspring of data.

And new information could in turn become an impetus to a new public awakening.

Back in the "early days," of course, lots of folks couldn't even recite the key signs of breast cancer — a lump or swelling in the breast, a discharge from the nipple other than breast milk, a redness or scales on the breast, or a pain in the nipple.

Many observers trace breast cancer consciousness to 1974, when then-First Lady Betty Ford publicized her diagnosis and mastectomy. But it took two decades before awareness became a political badge of honor.

A newspaper column in October 1995 by Hillary Rodham Clinton, who later would later run for president and serve as Secretary of State, pushed mammograms and noted, "One in eight women in our country will develop breast cancer during her lifetime, compared to one in 20 a generation ago."

Her husband, President Bill Clinton, shortly thereafter summoned images of his mother, dead from the disease, in an appeal for Congressional money to fight it. He also announced plans to shift $30 million into research on cancer-related genes.

Heartfelt altruism?

I figured his re-election drive rather than his mom's premature departure led to the largesse. In my mind's eye, the breast cancer and campaign bandwagons had gassed up at the same filling station.

But only a few more months passed before U.S. Sen. Barbara Boxer, who at the time lived but a couple of miles from us, had asked the Centers for Disease Control and Prevention to "conduct a serious and intensive inquiry into the [San Francisco Bay Area's] extraordinarily high breast cancer rate."

As the American consciousness inched forward, an unforeseen spin-off occasionally resulted.

When AOL banned the word breast from cyberspace because of its rules against the "use of obscene or vulgar language," corporate officials were instantly forced to overrule themselves. The reversal followed a barrage of protests, many emanating from breast cancer support groups.

"We have spent so many years trying to teach women that breast cancer is not something to be ashamed of [but something] they need to be able to talk about," an American Cancer Society executive committee member told the Associated Press. "I don't have any problem with AOL trying to keep dirty words off their service. But I don't consider breast to be a dirty word."

AOL inadvertently had turned the disease into a hot-button issue. Individual and business breast cancer activists couldn't wait to hop on the publicity train.

But no matter how fast public interest evolved, our private focus lingered on mortality issues.

Nance and I talked of cancer as seldom as possible yet, long after the treatments ended, people still asked, with a flat-line tone of apprehension, "How's Nance?" Though neither of us showed it, we were bothered by the question and its hidden agenda: "Has it returned?"

Then, one day during an especially challenging period, Nance tripped over her tongue. She meant to say "biopsy" but told me she was going to have an "autopsy."

I doubt if she'd heard herself. But — for what seemed an eternity — I froze.

Thankfully, her biopsy came back negative.

So did a subsequent one.

Both resulted from a purplish-reddish mark her masseuse found on Nance's side and back. It consisted of an oval, four inches in length and a couple of inches deep, with some hard stuff underneath.

We'd gone bonkers at the discovery.

Truthfully, nearly every time something out of kilter happened, our first reaction was to panic. Our second was to remember to breathe deeply.

We hardly stand alone in that regard. During one Man to Man session a newcomer slipped and referred to breast cancer as a "terminal disease." Another guy instantly jumped on him. "Life threatening, you mean," he said.

"Yeah, life threatening," said the first. But his voice lacked conviction.

Right after the masseuse discovered my wife's latest abnormality, Nance directed her dermatologist "to find out what it is no matter what it takes."

We were dissatisfied with the test results, which were inconclusive, so she visited her internist. He checked for Lyme's Disease and put her on an antibiotic as a preventive. Given that news, my partner admitted she was frantic. "I'm terrified that my immune system and body have been weakened so much by the cancer treatments I won't be able to fight a disease that difficult," she said.

"It would be ironic for me to have beaten cancer and then be killed by a tick."

Although tests eventually showed Nance *only* had arthritis, no doctor could pinpoint why the physically harmless mass and discoloration had appeared.

Unfortunately, my wife was tormented by the arthritis. Her hands ached. So did her face. She couldn't put weight on her knees. She had immense trouble gripping bottle tops, faucets, virtually anything at all. Rubbing had been no help. Heat had done nothing. Pain relievers were useless.

Her sciatica was getting worse, too.

She was convinced both arthritis and sciatica were a direct result of the chemo, her whipping boy anytime she needed one.

As those aches and pains kept her body and mind wobbly, hot flashes made her drip. "It's like walking into a furnace five times a day and standing there sweating for a minute and a half," she explained.

But sadness about her missing hair — even though that loss was temporary — remained the biggie for Nance. A year after her final treatment, she wrote in her journal that it *"was clearly the most psychologically devastating part of the cancer. It is still an issue for me.*

"My hair had been shoulder length and red and thick, a real signature, the one part of my body that I have loved unconditionally.

"I recently pulled my too-short-to-look-like-anything and too-long-to-style locks into a stub of a ponytail, and it felt cool, off my face, and neat. But it looked like shit: Its resemblance to a budding artichoke pasted to the top of my head was striking.

"I wasn't ready for going out in public this way, so I started thinking about alternatives and remembered that I had a hunk of hair, exactly the right color and length, tucked into my bureau. It was the hair that I'd had lopped off the day my hair started falling out from chemo. I rescued it from its nest, put it into an auburn hairnet, and plopped this bun on top of the cactus.

"It was magic. It looked great. The match, of course, was perfect, as was the texture. It easily fastened to my head with a few long hairpins, and I felt a lot like my old self.

"I had transformed the lemons, and was savoring the lemonade. I still am."

Be that as it may, on spotting a female punk with a shaved head shortly after making that entry, Nance thought: *"You dumb bitch, don't you know how lucky you are to have hair?"*

One thing's for sure, we agreed afterwards, absolutely everything's a matter of how you look at it.

And if Franklin Delano Roosevelt was right, we've never had anything to fear "but fear itself." Yet how many hundreds of times have we needed to invoke his words to ease our apprehension?

A study by the National Council on Aging showed more than 60 percent of older women in the United States were more afraid of cancer (especially breast cancer) than other disorders. And because of that angst, they might not take precautions against even bigger killers such as heart disease and stroke.

Death, it's clear, tends to be embraced most easily by true believers, those who totally buy into an afterlife.

When one of my support group members died by simply going to bed and forgetting to wake up, it upset the rest of us. We'd collectively worried about his wife but never given a second thought to *his* physical condition. There had been no reason to; on the surface, he seemed in tip-top health.

The unpredictability of life once more became a wake-up call, a directive to change perspective by adding a sweetener to our squeezed lemon juice.

"How long do any of us have?" The question racquet-balled off the walls of my brain. It became another reminder to live each day to the fullest, one at a time.

9

MEDS

The glut of ever-changing information about breast cancer drugs practically guarantees confusion for patients and caregivers, who are likely to be overwhelmed. New mainstream meds almost always seem appealing. But so do a lot of alternative treatments.

And the cancer industry's constant flip-flopping can be crazy-making.

The entire medical world, in fact, did a U-turn after 2002 findings that hormone-replacement therapy could lead to breast cancer.

The Women's Health Initiative study of 15,730 postmenopausal women clearly showed that those who'd had therapy combining estrogen and progestin faced a greater risk of getting the disease. The replacement therapy apparently also raised the chance of strokes, heart attacks and blood clots.

The cancer industry blanched.

And it took a full year for the FDA to insist manufacturers of meds with estrogen or an estrogen-progestin combo label them with appropriate warnings.

Trial results released in 2010 again raised red flags, this time that treatments combining estrogen and progestin could increase chances that an ensuing breast cancer could be fatal. And in 2012, a new study that tracked 60,000 nurses indicated that using any hormones for 10 years or longer could raise the breast cancer risk.

Nancy's oncologist had believed taking any of the steroid-hormone was a no-no. My wife's gynecologist had disagreed, though.

"Estrogen could not only ward off heart disease and osteoporosis," the latter said, "it could relieve vaginal dryness and thinning, insomnia and hot flashes."

In short, it might make Nance feel better, alleviate many of her side effects, and restore sexual desire and capability.

Which approach was correct for her?

Heaven only knew but, as it had since Ten Commandment days, remained silent. So we went with our instincts rather than desires, deciding if we were to err it should be on the side of caution and a lengthier life: We vetoed any use of estrogen (which, by the way, had received its original Federal Drug Administration approval as a treatment for menopause symptoms in the dinosaur days of Western medicine, 1942).

Today's news about medicines, or tomorrow's, assuredly can bring new awareness.

But overblown dispatches about cutting-edge pharmaceuticals, tests and treatments are also certain to create abject confusion.

Cancer researchers and the media long ago merged into a med-of-the-month club. Why? Sensational reports, even when premature, stimulate big headlines, sound bites or online flashes. They, in turn, sell newspapers or airtime or boost ratings. For scientists, that can translate into an influx of money to further their investigations.

In 2008, the Food and Drug Administration provided "accelerated approval" for Avastin, an angiostatin, to treat advanced breast cancer because the drug purportedly slowed down the progress of malignancies.

A handful of medics questioned whether the annual $96,000 cost of stifling cancer for a few months before it again ran wild was worth it.

But their voices were buried by news outlets feeding the inflated hopes of a public starved for a cure — even though no one claimed the drug bolstered survival rates.

Later, researchers at the University of California, San Francisco, voiced fears Avastin could inflame tumors and cause the spread of invasive growths to other body parts. And in 2010, the Associated Press noted that new studies showed the drug — which by then was being prescribed to some 17,500 women annually — failed to extend lives.

That December, the FDA recommended that Avastin no longer be used to treat breast cancer. And in late 2011 it officially revoked its approval for that purpose, the first time the agency had taken such a dramatic step.

Curiously, however, a government spokesman said Medicare would cover the drug for patients anyway.

Huh?

In 2012, two new studies (one in the United States, one in Germany) indicated the same drug might be effective in fighting early breast cancers. The research wasn't complete, though, so conclusions about survival were kept in the wings.

Just to complicate the issue, Genentech, its manufacturer, warned shortly afterwards that counterfeit vials were being made abroad and distributed in the United States in spite of the fakes missing a key ingredient.

All the back and forth, all the hem-and-hawing, about the best-selling cancer drug tended to replicate the history of other meds.

In 1998, a story in The New York Times was condemned widely for declaring that endostatin and angiostatin could "eradicate any type of cancer, with no obvious side effects and no drug resistance, in mice."

Critics charged the front-page piece romanticized the role of the researcher, Dr. Judah Folkman.

The National Cancer Institute joined the parade of vultures pecking at the bones of the paper. It cited 11 similar meds in clinical trials, including three at more advanced testing levels.

What had pushed the story over the top?

The Times had quoted molecular biologist James D. Watson, Nobel laureate who'd discovered the "double helix" structure of DNA, that "Judah is going to cure cancer in two years."

The experience of Nance's oncologist was typical: 80 percent of her patients asked if they should take either drug.

Or both.

As might have been predicted, a series of side effects swiftly came to light: loss of sensation in limbs, brain-cell toxicity, skeletal stiffness and muscle inflammation.

It's become obvious that each new breast cancer find, and every new application, needs to be wrapped in a massive question mark.

Consider tamoxifen.

The initial consensus: A "miracle drug" that could extend the life of many patients.

Few argued about its benefits. They'd been clearly outlined by a study of 37,000 patients based on a decade-and-a-half analysis of 55 trials in 15 countries. But some skeptics called the estrogen-suppressor highly dangerous, despite reports of a six-year National Cancer Institute study of 13,388 high-risk women showing it could cut chances of breast cancer recurrence almost in half.

Lo and behold, foes reported the drug had serious side effects: It doubled the risk for cancer in the uterine lining. It tripled the chances of blood clots in the lungs.

It also, incidentally, increased the odds of developing cataracts.

Women over 50 were touted as particularly vulnerable. For every 1,000 women in that age bracket with a uterus, tamoxifen reputedly prevented 20 breast cancers.

But caused 22 life-threatening complications.

Study results released in 2012, in sheer contrast, claimed "women should be taking the drug for twice as long as customary, a finding that could upend the standard that has been in place for about 15 years," according to The New York Times.

The revamped bottom line, extracted from a study of 7,000 women from three-dozen countries: A 10-year regimen of tamoxifen should be substituted for the 5-year treatment.

What, then, supposedly would happen? Recurrence and death rates might descend.

The drug debates were giving me a mental whiplash not unlike the impact of being rear-ended in a middle of a seven-car crash. And Nance's support group unanimously supported a member's pithy assertion that the pro/con seesaw came down to "all the reports having been sculpted out of a single pile of horseshit."

Need another drug-confusion illustration?

Newspapers throughout the country detailed two studies claiming raloxifene could cut the incidence of breast cancer by 50 percent — in the short run, anyway.

According to a survey of 19,000 postmenopausal women who took it an average of two years and five months, the med — which also blocked the action of estrogen and was sold under the brand name Evista — didn't raise the risk of uterine cancer as did tamoxifen.

Voila!

Another spanking new "wonder drug."

But it also, not unexpectedly, came with an assortment of side effects — among them leg cramps, hot flashes, a possible increase in water retention, deadly strokes and vein blood clots that could become fatal if they traveled to the lungs.

Its miracle-drug status, of course, didn't last longer than it took to ask someone in medical research circles, "Whazzup?"

I remember having blinked one morning only to find it had become Taxol's turn in the limelight.

The FDA had endorsed the med's use for patients with early-stage breast cancer, not long after the manufacturer had won federal approval to fight advanced breast cancer, ovarian cancer and some lung malignancies.

Yes, the drug had side effects, neurological tidbits like numbness of the hands and feet — but not to worry, the feds indicated, it'll be a valuable addition to your medicine cabinet.

"I'm up to my ears in information," I whined one afternoon, "and I'm sure I'd be half-crazed even if every damned study didn't challenge the previous one."

The jury's still out, for God-knows how lengthy a time, on eribulin, an experimental drug made from sea sponges.

One 2010 study suggested it could extend the lives of patients with advanced breast cancer. But researchers weren't scheduled to report on other trials for years.

It's amazing, of course, how breast cancer patients and partners absorb new data. It's amazing, too, how quickly we can develop an affinity for rodents, at least the lab kind.

My partner and I latched onto a copy of the journal Science promoting the notion that tumors in mice could be killed by engineered blood clots. The therapy, akin to killing a plant by cutting off its roots, reputedly caused cancer cells to die within a day. Tests on humans, unfortunately, were light years away.

The bottom line: Any given news item might be a momentous step forward for the little critters, not so much for humanity.

But human hope is a wondrous thing to stash in your back pocket.

Take, for example, Zometa, a drug given intravenously for cancers that have spread to the bones.

In 2009, the New England Journal of Medicine predicted the benefits of the med some day might equal those of chemo or hormonal therapy. And in 2011, a seven-year study indicated it improved breast cancer survival, dropping the risk of death by 37 percent.

Hot damn!

But in 2014, when I googled for an update, I found a post by a San Francisco advocacy group, Breast Cancer Action, that was largely critical of a luncheon presentation by Zometa's manufacturer, Novartis. The organization, in effect, had questioned the drug's merit — and the company's P.R. thrust.

The piece concluded that the "well informed, passionate...activists and advocates [who attended wanted] real information, not pablum sugar-coated."

I readily admit that because Nance and I tend to be right-brained, we're a lot more apt to check out the less-technical news stories. Such as those that described cancer patients warding off pain via a raspberry-flavored "narcotic lollipop."

Actiq, a prescriptive drug, hypothetically could flow into the bloodstream faster than any pill — although the good-tasting sucker might cause nausea, constipation and dizziness. Detractors also charged that the FDA-approved painkiller was a risk to kids who might be lured into fatal usage.

Meanwhile, though conventional Western medicine remained the biggest weapon on Nance's munitions rack, it was hardly her only one — even though alternative practitioners had few or no governmental safeguards.

Of the many supplementary modalities and healers utilized in search of a cure, she'd located a local practitioner of Chinese medicine who still ranks high. My wife's belief in him is totally practical:

If what he suggests doesn't hurt her, why not try it?

It's evident she's had nothing to lose except a relatively insignificant amount of cash.

After the surgical, radiation and chemo treatments had finished, he recommended she start a new regimen in addition to the COQ10 gel and thymic compound he'd previously advocated.

The list included DHA oil, a fatty acid to bolster the cardiovascular system; alpha lipoic acid and another seasonal anti-oxidant; mushroom combination caps, an immune-enhancer and mild liver cleanser; plus a calcium capsule, natural vitamin E and a bio-enhanced multiple vitamin.

As surely as I would stumble over pronunciations, Nance planned to "follow his guidance."

I'm confident that if she'd believed munching on snakeskin would prevent a recurrence, she'd have chomped away. And, to be honest, I would probably have applauded her action.

But please understand: I reside in California, a state (or state of mind, if you will) that non-politically correct name-callers assure us "is the land of fruits and nuts." And if someone were seeking an unconventional modus operandi for healing, well, my home county expressly embraces quirky.

Need a specific or two?

Well, peek at the Marin-based Tamalpa Institute's "creative response to the breast cancer crisis." One flyer spotlighted a sweat-lodge ceremony for women, an art exhibit "featuring psycho-kinetic drawings by people facing cancer," and "an opportunity to deepen our experience of the planetary dance."

In our neck of the woods, alternative healing methods gain adherents faster than Moonies can marry.

Marin General Hospital at various times established acupuncture and massage programs as well as "integrative oncology," an individualized treatment that featured jin shin jyutsu ("an ancient Japanese art of longevity, benevolence and happiness"), and classes in yoga, tai chi and qi gong.

But while Nance and many of her support group pals generally favored testing fresh or even untried ideas, clinical drug trials were decidedly an experiment of a different color.

Patients couldn't distance themselves fast enough.

Some laid blame on potential side effects. But it appeared clear to my wife and me that the women, even in advanced stages of breast cancer, didn't want to chance any further deterioration of their quality of life.

Still another factor in not volunteering, Nance and I theorized, was pure exhaustion with the healing process.

In fact, when I asked about the possibilities of her helping out, she whimpered, "I can't, I just can't. I've gone through too many tests and treatments already."

Appears to be a widespread posture.

A report from the National Cancer Institute gloomily stipulated that only 3 percent of eligible breast cancer patients across the country had participated in an extensive sampling of trials.

No matter: New approaches, treatments and meds for breast cancer — like Energizer bunnies escaping from their hutch — just keep on keepin' on.

An international study discovered Femara (estrogen-lowering drugs in the aromatase-inhibitor class, along with Arimidex and Aromasin) might fight advanced breast cancer better than tamoxifen.

The survey of 907 postmenopausal females found it let women put off more toxic chemo for several months.

Although years and years of additional testing were anticipated for the trio of meds, even the first examination of Arimidex (aka anastrozole), a five-year test of 4,500 postmenopausal women, 2,000 of them healthy, had been dogged by controversy over giving experimental medication to patients who were well.

Part of the reason for the flap was that it came with such side effects as high blood pressure, fatigue and hot flashes.

And while tests for Aromasin, also called exemestane, had shown it apparently had fewer side issues, it reportedly did cause more bone-thinning, joint pain and diarrhea.

Despite the hopes raised by all three meds, Baylor College of Medicine academics hoisted a novel warning sign for patients: Laboratories were using arbitrary standards — which deviated from lab to lab, and even from pathologist to pathologist in the same hospital — when testing estrogen receptors. Because of those vacillating measures, thousands of women might mistakenly reject tamoxifen, the report charged.

The only constant, it seemed, was that scientific thought processes (much like my belt size) needed nonstop adjusting.

Drugs obviously wax and wane in popularity — among patients and medical professionals.

In 2013, for example, the FDA approved Kadcyla, a new "conjugate drug" that links — according to an article in The New York Times — "to proteins known as monoclonal antibodies" (also known, in the case of breast cancer, as HER2), which in turn latch onto tumors but spare healthy cells and dodge some side effects.

It was pricey: $94,000 for an average course (about $10,000 per month), double the charge for Herceptin, a previously best-selling breast cancer med that was incorporated in the new one.

But six months of life supposedly could be added to a late-stage patient whose cancer has metastasized, though the drug's list of potential side effects is rather lengthy. Which, logically, brings up to need for a patient to weigh her quality of life against her life expectancy.

Finally, if the information within this chapter frazzles you, know you're not alone. It indeed can be, plainly put, daunting.

And time is only likely to increase its complexity.

Do know, however, that if your partner intends to use any of the drugs mentioned, you both would do well to go backwards for a moment — and reflect on a fundamental question posed when the 2002 U-turn occurred: Is estrogen a life-expanding gift or a source of breast cancer?

Scientists had decided, in virtually the same breath they'd been praising estrogen treatments, that the chemical should be added to the nation's list of cancer-causing agents. A National Institutes of Health advisory board voted to warn patients but not ban it because, despite its hazards, it might cut out debilitating menopausal symptoms.

About 16 million postmenopausal women had been using hormone replacement therapy at that juncture — solo estrogen or in conjunction with progestin.

Ignorance, ostensibly, had long been the hidden ingredient in birth-control pills.

It undoubtedly had been common knowledge the quickie portal to recreational sex carried a dash of estrogen. But what few later wanted to cop to was the idea that women with a family history of breast cancer who'd taken pre-1975 pills (which had much higher levels of the hormone than today's) had acquired a substantially higher risk of the disease along with their sexual freedom.

OMG!

The human ostriches naively had preferred to ignore scientific evidence The Pill could increase the odds of getting breast cancer more than 50 percent if the taker was over the age of 45 — a chilling statistic that leapt from a massive study of 103,027 Norwegian and Swedish women.

By the time those findings were released, of course, Nance, who'd been taking them for decades, was miles beyond fretting about birth-control pills.

10

AS YEARS GO BY

During my wife's treatments, we couldn't escape the speeding highs and lows of the cancer coaster any more than toddlers can slay the fierce dragons lurking under their beds or in their closets. By the five-year point after Nancy's treatments, we'd managed to quash most of the unpleasant memories, though a few hangers-on continued to gnaw at us. I suspect that, barring an absolute onslaught of Alzheimer's, we'll never completely shed the frayed psychological overcoats of yesterday.

"I have daily reminders of the illness," she wrote in her journal, *"that make it impossible for me to forget it all.*

"The back of my right arm is still totally numb, and the feeling will probably never return. My right nipple is a pale pink, compared to the deeper shade of my left. I have arthritis in my hands and feet, which ache constantly; I relieve it slightly with a daily dose of Aleve.

"My vagina still needs regular lubrication, and my sex drive, diminished though it was even before the cancer, has virtually disappeared.

"I have scars on my chest; 20 extra pounds from cookies I ate to make me feel better; wiry, erect chin hairs that replace themselves nightly like amoebas in a frenzied state of asexual reproduction; thick, red-white hair that's still 'growing in.'

"I also have no hair under both my arms, despite that fact that the radiation was only on one side. I don't miss the hair but I wonder what other 'hidden parts' died and won't come back.

"None of this physical stuff is 'awful.' Most of it, I tell myself, 'should be the worst thing that ever happens to me.' Some of it is a constant annoyance, an irritating drip on my head, a Chinese water-torture of sorts that keeps my brain

aware that I'm a survivor.

"I begin and end each day with a huge handful of antioxidents, vitamin supplements, thymus, COQ10 and other capsules designed to pump up my system and make me feel good so I'll age and age and age.

"I used to dread aging. Now I'm grateful to have that privilege."

I could fully relate to that last paragraph. I wasn't thrilled with the slow degeneration that accompanies the graying process, but I definitely viewed Nancy's dyeing a vastly better option than her dying.

My partner's tresses had eventually reached a length she was comfortable with, although she needed three haircuts within a week to get it right. The stylist was ultra-conservative, afraid to trim too much after having watched her go through the entire painful losing-and-growing process.

Nance's hair came back thick and course, strangely different than its former soft texture. A slight wave still broke, but all the curls had vanished.

Both of us were positive the changes were preferable to no hair.

It had taken more than two years before she could look at images of her baldness, however. She agreed at last to put the photos of her hairless stage into two albums.

"Wow, was I ever ugly," she declared.

Her words triggered my caregiver button. "You and I will never see it the same way," I replied sincerely. "Your high cheekbones and eyes showed off better when there was no hair to look at. The fact is, you're lovely both ways."

Said she: "Boy, was I ever unattractive."

I have no trouble recalling precisely when the re-growth began — I'd playfully called her Stubblehead. She felt ambivalent, disliking the name but loving the idea new hair was coming in. And she couldn't wait to tint it back to her original color.

While Nancy had worried about her follicles, I fretted about something else.

I'd viewed a 20-minute American Cancer Society video, "A Significant Journey," subtitled "Breast Cancer Survivors and the Men Who Love Them." It bothered me the documentary, as most literature and audio-visual aids on the subject, adhered to a female point of view: Males apparently were considered semi-useful appendages.

When I told my men's group about it, each guy empathized.

"Women, of course, are the ones whose lives are being threatened. It's natural they get the biggest share of attention and sympathy," one regular noted. "But I would like just a little bit of those things."

The nods of assent showed the feeling to be unanimous.

Simpatico sentiments have been commonplace within the group, where fellowship stems from all of us paddling to keep the same boat afloat. We couldn't care less if what we said was clichéd, trite, worn-out. For the most part, our rambling conversations lifted us.

But every once in a while, one member's melancholy could turn an entire gathering sour.

A young guy told us, with colossal regret, he felt forced to abandon the San Francisco Bay Area because of the high cost of maintenance. He simply couldn't handle the bills, even with insurance covering a large percentage.

Most patients and caregivers ignore the costs of cancer at first; they're too immersed in the disease itself. But then, like a clap of thunder, the financial burden strikes out of nowhere. Each attendee at one time or another has been forced to battle toe-to-toe with insurance companies — as well as with that monster side-effect of breast cancer, dread.

I wasn't immune to either.

Negative input particularly overwhelmed me during one "week from hell" in which a member's sister, who'd already lost an eye to melanoma, suffered a stroke, and another's wife unexpectedly started to fail.

My mortality and my wife's lay across my chest like a smug 320-pound National Football League defensive lineman who'd just made a crucial tackle.

I found it hard to exhale. It helped to talk openly about it.

It had been a long time since I'd thought I needed support. I'd slipped easily into the role of Man to Man's main contact person when a founder of the group who was moving to another state urged me to replace him as point person. From that moment on, I'd mistakenly believed I'd no doubt be the one dispensing advice based on my personal experience, not receiving it.

Wrong!

I'd made another misstep, albeit momentary, too. After several years of regularly attending the weekly meetings, I casually mentioned to Nance that I occasionally became phlegmatic.

She jumped on my comment and asked why, if that were accurate, I continued to go. I thought for about a second and a quarter. "It's critically important," I said sotto voce, "even if no newbie shows up this week, next week, next month or in six months. We need to be there *whenever* somebody needs help."

Nance's question/ploy had prompted exactly the response she expected.

She also knew that many parallels existed between the men's gatherings and the women's.

Both, for example, were poised virtually every second to laugh at the teeniest bit of humor. Case in point: An oldtimer's wife fell and cut her head. Although there was no connection to her cancer, she managed to carve an oblique link. Her sole comment, walking into the emergency room, was, "Oh, no, not *another* fucking scar."

Buoyant items sometimes jumped out of the ozone.

A regular whose wife had died informed us about his new romance. It had blossomed in a grief group.

His report pleased us all, although as a unit we flashed back to how difficult it had been for him the previous year. His spouse's final journey had been slow and painful.

He'd invited everyone in the group, and our partners, to her memorial service.

In the back yard, handholding relatives and acquaintances formed a ring in which the cancer victim's daughter sang sweetly. A woman sitting under a tree just beyond the circle was breast-feeding her infant.

Nance was agitated by the memorial.

"Rarely was his wife treated as a full human being in the service," she noted later. "Only once was her anger mentioned, only once was her disgust with the medical establishment referred to. Her pain and suffering were talked about but usually in a context of how she dealt courageously with it. Not once did anyone say she was so drugged on morphine at the end she wasn't here. And no one mentioned she made peace with her mother but had a lifelong series of difficulties with her.

"Why do we make saints of the dead? Why don't we let them remain human?"

She paused, then added: "Throughout the service I kept thinking that she has left this plane, that I could have been the woman who died after a year and a half's painful cancer deterioration."

I later realized Man to Man members normally don't display pictures of our partners or describe any parts of them except for diseased boobs. I'd never met the guy's dead wife. When she passed on, I was unable to visualize her. Only after I saw her photograph in their home did she become real to me.

"That's really bizarre," I'd thought. "She had to die before I could see her as being alive."

A few weeks after the memorial, Nance and I fought about something trivial just before I left for a group breakfast. She jolted me with her parting remark: "I'm privileged to be able to argue," she said. "Some breast cancer patients can't — they're dead."

More typically, she — and I and members of both support groups — stayed upbeat by, as the classic song lyric spells out, accentuating the positive.

But her peers occasionally risked stepping onto a down escalator by discussing such nuisances as cancer-cure sensationalism: "We're always hopeful a breast cancer breakthrough will occur but we are very cautious," Nance reported. "There's always momentary optimism when the media go crazy, but we're also aware they'll make something sound like a cure-all when it isn't. Several women emphasized that what works in mice doesn't always work in humans."

She specifically cited tamoxifen, which had been taken by several in her group, as a poignant sampling. "What the media neglected to do was mention all the side effects, of which we're so keenly aware."

To prevent my thinking her group stressed anything other than living, my spouse then listed some joyful changes breast cancer had prompted.

One woman bought a new home. Another overhauled her life to get credentials for a new profession. A third quit her job and become a part-time volunteer.

"We talk in the group about losing the sense of immortality, about how there is only now," Nance said.

The prism through which she and I most often view "now" has become multi-colored, like a field of wildflowers. Bright. She has survived. So have I. When we reached the five-year mark, we felt as if we'd conquered breast cancer, our terrors and the rollercoaster.

But a dispatch in the Marin Independent Journal had momentarily shaken us from that tranquility. It showed our home county's breast cancer rate rising dramatically.

Speculation swiftly became the local game of the week, with blame falling on, well, you name it: Women here being better educated, being better off financially, having no children or having them later in life, and being Caucasian.

The speculative flip-flop continued unabated for years.

In late 2012, new research found four breast cancer clusters in California, including Marin, but it offered no clues as to why rates were higher in those areas. And in 2013, statewide figures pinpointed Marin's rates at 20 percent higher than the national average.

The good news, based on 2006-10 stats, was that mortality rates were dropping — though the reasons for the dip remained unclear.

Across the country, the director of the Silent Spring Institute in Newton, Mass., another nesting community for the disease, had been busily faulting common items that contain chemicals known to speed the growth of malignant cells — laundry detergent, food packaging, plastic toys, disinfectants, spermicidal and synthetic hormones, synthetic leather, insect repellents and pesticides.

It appeared likely, however, that our wealthy county's mystery would remain unsolved — until a Man to Man attendee defused the fear with a touch of levity. "The cause is the environment in upscale Marin," he said with a sheepish grin. "It's from the magnetic strips on so many credit cards."

Clearly, today's fact can convert into tomorrow's fiction.

The local breast cancer rate became a perfect model for that truism when the National Cancer Institute deflated the notion that it was one of the worst in the country. After reviewing census data, it determined our rate was in line with other California areas and just a bit above the national average.

My restless mind then darted to my files. They were jammed with statistics, charts, data, death rates, cure rates. Each had made at least a temporary dent in my thinking.

But I chided myself for forgetting the breast cancer coaster is not exactly a modern, electric-powered vehicle. It is, rather, an old-fashioned gas-and news-guzzler — one fueled by an incessant fusillade of items delivered on deadlines that often preclude fact-checking by print-journalists, bloggers and assorted denizens of the internet, as well as TV and radio anchors.

Newscasts, despite my occupation, not infrequently made me edgy.

I'd mentioned that to my shrink. She suggested that I find a way to change my attitude, to focus more on the positive.

She also suggested that Nance and I were "still both needy right now and should figure out how to take turns nurturing."

Support, she also helped me recognize, is a necessity not merely for cancer patients and prime caregivers but for siblings and those in the next generation.

Though my wife and I had internalized our disappointment in her daughter for what we considered insufficient support during the breast cancer treatments, an insight belatedly bubbled up: Neither Nance nor I had tried to help her face the terror she was going through when her mom's life was being threatened.

When it came to my own alarms, I'd frequently invoked my favorite feel-good, lift-me-by-the-bootstraps standby homily, "I wept because I had no shoes, and then I met a man who had no feet."

It usually calmed me down.

And it had helped me look at other breast cancer patients who were — or had been — worse off than Nance. Or at partners who'd had a tougher road to repave than I.

I'd also leaned on the Talmudic at various times: "If I am not for myself, who will be for me? But if I am only for myself, what am I?"

That had allowed me to re-focus on why I remained in the support group.

If I were wriggling in emotional quicksand that threatened to drag me under, however, my best credo had become the biblical edict that promoted patience: "And this, too, shall pass."

For sure, my reality would be 100 percent spectacular if I could look at each detail of my life and change it for the better simply by applying a homily — or if I could turn any moment of crisis into a memento, or cling to a cerebral talisman. Or if I'd take a little more time out to smell the fragrant Stargazer lilies I buy for Nance each week.

But regardless how many mottos or bouquets I've been armed with, or how hard I'd try, I just couldn't stay positive day in and day out.

Nance had accidentally pushed my panic button one day when I piled a six-month reserve of toilet paper onto a Costco shopping cart. She called it "a lifetime supply." My dread and anger had instantly merged into a single unwarranted explosion.

"I don't want you ever to imply a truncated lifetime, even in an attempt at humor," I shouted.

Trailing the blow-up came a vulnerable, guilt-bloated apology. "I'm still scared your lifetime could be shortened without warning," I admitted.

The looming face of death can be creepy. It can even disillusion those who have studied it extensively and are supposedly ready. A seriously ailing 70-year-old Elizabeth Kubler-Ross, who'd written the classic book "On Death and Dying," was so angry about her condition she rejected her own worth — and God's — and declared her life's work had been for nothing.

Many in her coterie needed to take the time to tell her repeatedly she was wrong, she *had* helped.

Everyone except a teenager racing 130 mph in a souped-up Mustang normally acknowledges death is unavoidable. For the rest of us, minions of the Grim Reaper can lurk around a corner least expected.

On the other hand, death can also become a catalyst for living.

So can impending death.

Lisa Bonchek Adams, according to a story in The Guardian in 2014, was dying a painful death of breast cancer that had spread "to her bones, joints, hips, spine, liver and lungs." She blog-tweeted about her journey hundreds of thousands of times, starting each day with the same thought: "Find a bit of beauty in the world today. Share it. If you can't find it, create it. Some days this may be hard to do. Persevere."

I certainly wasn't dying, but I still wasn't immune to death thoughts.

My thirty-something son had found himself in a quandary. His words were few, his archetypical question anything but simple: "What should I do with my life?"

His reverie was triggered by his divorce from a movie chain for which he'd run multiplex theaters in Florida and Georgia. My son, who for nearly a decade had tinkered with the idea of starting his own business, wanted to buy into a coupon-publication franchise. My reaction? Unadulterated ambivalence.

I believed it would take him years to make a meaningful profit, and that he'd be dissatisfied with the low level of income the business would generate before then. At the same time, I wanted to encourage his quest for independence.

From God's country came my answer. The 32-year-old husband of my former assistant dropped dead. Heart attack.

My phone carrier couldn't connect me fast enough. "Go ahead and do it," I said. "If you're going to take some big risks, or make any big mistakes, now's the time. Don't wait until you're too old to ward off the punches."

He knew I'd been unsure so he didn't understand how my position had solidified so quickly. I told him of the death.

"Don't wait," I repeated. "You can never be sure there'll be a tomorrow."

11

RESEARCH

Researchers in the cancer industry flip-flop almost as often as presidential candidates do.

Regulars in Man to Man (as well as in Nancy's support group) were of a single mind: If any individual study proved X, as sure as the sun would come up the next day, there'd soon be a survey that specified Y was true.

But for argument's sake, let's imagine something virtually unimaginable: Doctors and researchers can collectively agree on an issue.

The truth is, such accord does exist — at least as of 10:28 a.m. today, the moment this is being written — in the form of a belief that most women with breast cancer are likely to do as well with lumpectomies as with single or double mastectomies.

No one should hold his or her breath, however; in a week or two, or a minute or two, there may be a complete reversal.

Medical professionals who advocated removing only the cancerous mass had inched into a majority position by the tail of the 20th century. Before 1985, however, the lumpectomy couldn't gain much traction; the mastectomy, introduced nearly 100 years earlier, had remained the standard.

Not that long ago a study outlined in the Journal of the American Medical Association found early breast cancer tumors had often been "over-treated." Translation: Radical breast removal wasn't necessary.

And two subsequent studies found, when cancers were comparatively small, lumpectomies plus radiation equal to mastectomy over a 10-year period.

Had the research ended there, few doubts would have arisen. But medical explorations don't seem ever to stop.

Subsequent conclusions in the New England Journal of Medicine reasoned that women who'd had only a lumpectomy were three times more apt to suffer a recurrence than those who'd had the surgery and radiation.

Thus, as informed patients and partners might guess, the healing pendulum began hurtling back and, for a while, mastectomies again became the treatment du jour.

A Mayo Clinic study underscored the swing of the treatment pendulum.

It noticed that prophylactic bilateral mastectomy of women with family histories of the disease had become increasingly widespread even when patients were healthy. Fear was the major impetus for the surgery — despite Canadian researchers claiming women who'd undergone the operation had "an exaggerated perception" of their peril.

The renewed thrust toward mastectomies also emanated from surgeons pushing reconstruction.

At first they used tissue from a patient's abdomen, forcing it upward and reshaping it into the form of a breast. But medics then honed a whole series of techniques, most popular of which became an operation called the Tram-flap. For many who did go through with reconstruction, though, life somehow failed to transform into a rose garden. Some complained of a loss of feeling in the areas that had been cut up; others griped their breasts ended up lopsided.

Regardless, the medical profession's overview on mastectomy and lumpectomy changed almost as frequently as its theories once had as to whether infants should be breast-fed or bottle-fed.

"Do you think I should have a preventive mastectomy?" Nance had asked me early on.

"I can't make that kind of decision for you," I'd replied, more than a little uncomfortable with her query, "but I always think the most conservative, least aggressive surgery is the best way to go."

"I guess I think that, too," she said.

We'd opted for the lumpectomy — and, happily, never really looked back.

A study of 112,154 women with early-stage breast cancer, released in 2013, apparently confirmed the wisdom of that decision: Having a lumpectomy followed by radiation resulted in a better survival rate than having a mastectomy (6 to 14 percent better, with results on the top end of the scale for women 50 years old and up).

Tangentially, the Mayo Clinic in 2014 reported research showing its team approach worked. Its system dictated the presence of a pathologist who'd freeze and slice tumors while a lumpectomy patient was still on the operating table. Clinicians maintained the process could reduce, from between 15 and 40 percent to a mere 3 percent, the chances of *not* finding escaped cancer cells that might later require a second surgery to "clear the margins," a procedure that helps ensure a patient being cancer-free.

Medical debates have hardly been limited to lumpectomy vs. mastectomy, however. The question of when — or even if — to use mammography, for example, is still being tossed about like a dingy in a hurricane.

Annual screenings for females in their 50s and 60s had won almost universal approval of physicians. By the turn of the 21st century, yearly mammograms for women in their 40s also were being supported by the American Medical Association, the American Cancer Society, the American College of Surgeons and the National Cancer Institute — in spite of dissent by the U.S. Preventative Services Task Force and the NCI's parent group, the National Institutes of Health.

Although mammography was long considered the first line of defense, arguably the best way of detecting breast cancer early, a slew of medics and researchers started to question if the procedure was sufficiently accurate.

Fears about excessive false-positives snowballed.

Some of the apprehension could be traced to research at Harvard and Washington universities that half those who had 10 mammograms would be given at least one wrong report of abnormalities.

That research also showed women who underwent annual mammograms after age 40 with a 19 percent chance of getting an unnecessary biopsy.

And the American College of Physicians, which represents 120,000 internists, issued guidelines saying females in their 40s should check with their doctors rather than automatically get mammograms — because the risks might outweigh the benefits.

Industry inside-outing turned into a full-fledged medical firestorm in 2009 following release of a federally funded report that suggested women in their 40s might not need mammograms at all. But those "new" guidelines, in reality, were almost identical to the task force's position of the 1990s. And the controversy replicated debates sparked by reports on the first large-scale trials of mammography in 1971.

It's unlikely the controversy will ever disappear.

In late 2012 a blue-ribbon British panel determined that although screenings for women over 50 did save lives, three women were over-diagnosed for each one saved.

That panel, which studied trials in Britain, the U.S., Canada and Sweden, claimed the over-diagnoses led to substantial harm — via chemo, surgery or radiation — to women whose cancers would never be dangerous.

Around that same time, according to the Associated Press, a U.S. study concluded that a third of women diagnosed with breast cancer over a 28-year period wouldn't have developed the disease had they been left alone, with more than a million women unnecessarily treated. The survey also showed the increasing use of mammograms had done little to decrease the death rate.

Nance and I sided with those who advocated screening, and believed cost paring was the main reason cutbacks were being pushed. We figured even a single life saved was worth some invasive procedures on other women.

In the meantime, some medical practitioners began spouting breast thermography as an alternative to mammograms.

In mid-2014, a study of 454,850 screenings suggested that a new test, tomosynthesis, often called 3-D mammography (because the machine moves around the breast), could decrease false alarms while stepping up the detection rate. The equipment, whose use was approved in the U.S. three years before, costs about $500,000, double that of a conventional digital mammography machine.

No matter what profits or politics intruded, or what any given patient, caregiver or pundit believed, my wife and I were convinced humor could overcome most misgivings when it came to breast cancer.

We both smiled, for example, at an anonymous "Ode to a Mammogram" someone had faxed to my office during Nance's treatment:

My skin was stretched 'n' stretched
From way up by my chin,
And my poor tit was being squashed
To Swedish-pancake thin.
If I had no problem when I came in,
I surely have one now.
If there had been a cyst in there,
It would have popped — ker-pow.
This machine was made by man;
Of this, I have no doubt.
I'd like to get his balls in there;
For months he'd go without.

Susan Love, a pioneer in breast cancer research, isn't known primarily for her sense of humor. She's famed, instead, as the expert on breast cancer — and she strongly believes in mammograms.

Love wrote what became the bible for my wife's intractable disease and its treatment — not unlike what Dr. Benjamin Spock had done with child rearing. Every diagnosed woman I knew had at least dipped into, or sworn by, "Dr. Susan Love's Breast Book," which first was published in 1990 and has since gone into a fifth edition.

Her extremely dense tome, which many found to be more useful as an encyclopedic reference work rather than a read-through, helped Nance and me more times than we can remember.

And while conventional wisdom insisted monthly self-exams could save a woman's life, Love ardently disagreed, referring to the belief as "wishful thinking." Self-exams are instead a foundation for psychological harm, she charged, saying her experience confirmed most women don't do it but feel guilty they don't.

True early detection, Love elaborated for the benefit of Newsweek and Parade readers, is something only mammograms can do — that is, find a tumor that's too small to feel.

All things considered, she kept on being optimistic.

She predicted in another Newsweek article, "We may well have a vaccine in my lifetime, gene therapy for women with a genetic susceptibility to the disease, or other tools more effective and benign than the 'slash, burn and poison' approach of surgery, radiation and chemotherapy."

The unvarnished truth, in my opinion, is that anyone who was — or is — looking for a quick fix or an irrefutable answer about anything related to breast cancer is on a bumpy road to disappointment.

It also might be safe to say that *everything* causes cancer. Or that ordinary living instigates it.

One study showed women who eat well-done beef and bacon have a four times greater chance of getting breast cancer than those who ate rare or medium meat.

Predictably, multiple analysts disagreed — without hesitation. They claimed, conversely, that undercooked meat posed the verifiable health risk. But they also admitted there was too much factual fuzziness for anyone to recommend everlasting changes in cooking habits.

Desire more debate fodder?

A trio of studies claimed, respectively, that heavy drinking significantly increases risk of the disease, women with dense breasts get cancer five times more than those with the most fatty tissue, and a link exists between intensified exposure of artificial lighting and breast cancer.

Needless to say, the medical juries are still deliberating.

Western medicine's harshest skeptics say it's foolish to depend on *any* research, breast cancer statistics or hotlines.

According to a piece in The New York Times, U.S. investigators reported nearly one-third of those who called a federal toll-free number for cancer information got a busy signal or hung up because they had to wait too long.

That story also said computerized databases listing clinical trials contained "incomplete, incorrect and outdated information."

It further noted one in five callers were referred to local hospitals, hospices, home health-care agencies, pain clinics, genetic counselors and providers of social services even though information on those community services was often inaccurate.

It may be a bit too easy to lay blame for everything that's wrong at government's doorstep, though.

And it's also unrealistic to condemn the environment — in spite of some research classifying that as breast cancer's root cause.

Scientific reports from the Massachusetts-based Silent Spring Institute claimed more than 200 commonly used chemicals cause breast cancer in animals. The most widespread are elements in shampoos and detergents, vehicle exhaust, fried foods, carpeting, adhesives, foam cushions and bedding, furniture polish and fabric cleaner.

In comparison, the New England Journal reported an ongoing Nurses' Health Study that demonstrated lingering traces of DDT and PCBs in the environment did *not* trigger breast cancer.

And a 2011 study by researchers at the California Pacific Medical Center in San Francisco said everyday consumer products, BPA (bisphenol A), which exists in food packaging and cans, and methylparaben, found in cosmetics, might kill the effectiveness of tamoxifen.

A major 270-page national report in 2013 suggested more money must be spent on studying environmental factors.

But when all the research arguments are in hand, what really produces the disease, and what should be done about it?

The answers are probably as multi-faceted as Sigmund Freud's theories.

Way back in the '90s, a joint Israeli and American study of 858 Ashkenazi Jews, those with ancestors from Central or Eastern Europe, had rocked that ethnic community. The research concluded that a small percentage contained a genetic abnormality that could increase their chances of getting breast or ovarian cancer.

A second study — detailed in the Nature Genetics journal — then showed a second defect in the same population grouping also promoted breast cancer.

Only one in 40 to 50 apparently carried one or both genes, which became known as BRCA1 and BRCA2 (abbreviations for BReast CAncer gene 1 and 2). But the mutations supposedly raised the cancer risk as high as 87 percent.

The upshot? More than a few Jewish women become so terrified they had both breasts removed as a prophylactic measure.

Relatives of those with the defect also worried.

A 2007 study claimed they were up to five times more likely to develop the disease, even if they didn't have the mutation, than women unrelated to carriers. In late 2011, a new study totally contradicted those findings. There's no added risk at all, it said. And the following year Stanford researchers announced a new online tool based on mathematical probabilities that could predict what will happen to women with BRCA1 or 2, whether they opt for a mastectomy or not.

Oscar-winning actress Angelina Jolie wrote an op-ed piece for The New York Times in 2013 in which the 37-year-old disclosed she'd had a preventive double mastectomy because she carried the BRCA1 gene. The mastectomies, she said, reduced her chances of developing breast cancer to under 5 percent.

She also had reconstruction and implant surgery.

In the op-ed, she paid homage to her "partner, Brad Pitt, who is so loving and supportive," then added, "So to anyone who has a wife or girlfriend going through this, know that you are a very important part."

The more studies and decisions Nance and I looked at, the clearer it became that breast cancer is such an extremely complicated issue its cause is unlikely to be monolithic.

We also figured the causes are about as impossible to pinpoint as locating weapons of mass destruction in Iraq was.

To all intents and purposes, every expert appeared to have an individually distinct opinion about the disease's origins. Take heredity as a for-instance.

San Francisco Focus magazine quoted a National Cancer Institute bio-statistician as saying that the most important factor "is family history." If breast cancer has struck your mother, sister or daughter, "your risk is about double the national average," the expert said unequivocally. "Breast cancer in two or more close relatives boosts it even more."

And yet, the magazine text acknowledged, "About three-quarters of women who develop breast cancer have no family history of cancer."

Simultaneously, studies presented at an American Cancer Society science-writers seminar showed, according to a story in USA Today, "daughters and sisters of women with breast cancer vastly overestimate their own risk of cancer, and are prone to depression." Most, the piece proclaimed, "believed they were 'doomed' to develop breast cancer, even when their actual risk was only slightly higher than normal."

And according to a survey by the National Breast Cancer Coalition, what a majority of women consider knowledge about the illness is frequently more mythology than fact.

The president of the coalition told the Chicago Tribune there's a belief that — despite no scientific evidence to back up the idea — eating enough fruits and veggies can prevent breast cancer. She also cited the erroneous notion that heredity causes most cases of the disease when, in actual fact, only 5 to 10 percent come from inherited genetic mutations.

The disease appears on no branch of Nance's family tree. That detail didn't stop her from contracting it.

False information is rampant, perhaps more today because blogs keep proliferating. And, yes, it may be basic human nature to cling to bad news rather than good. Maybe that's why so many patients and partners have ignored a "Mayo Clinic Guide to Women's Cancers" that listed five items — antiperspirants, under-wire bras, coffee, large breasts and breast implants — as having no significance regarding breast cancer risk.

What lies ahead? The same as what lies behind: Research, research and more research — about anything and everything.

Many findings, history shows, will collide with other material.

A survey of 100,000 U.S. nurses a few years back discovered women who'd had as few as three alcoholic drinks a week elevated their risk of developing breast cancer.

Shortly thereafter, a Daily Mail story reported findings of a University of Cambridge study of 13,525 women with breast cancer that a daily glass of wine could raise the survival rates of females with breast cancer as much as 20 percent — contradicting, naturally, a slew of earlier research labeling alcohol as one of the leading causes of the disease among healthy women.

Then, in 2013, new information said even one drink a day can put a woman at risk for hormone-receptor-positive breast cancer and other cancers. How? By hiking levels of estrogen and other chancy hormones.

Only a couple of months later, however, yet another survey claimed that moderate drinking may have zero impact on survival rates — and might even help.

In 2014, scientists at the University of California, San Diego, School of Medicine, reported breast cancer patients with high levels of vitamin D in their blood were twice as likely to survive the disease as women with low levels.

An earlier piece in the American Journal of Clinical Nutrition, itemizing a 10-year Swedish study that followed 35,000 women between the ages of 49 and 83, found those who took daily multi-vitamins were 19 percent more likely to develop breast cancer.

Factual? Even that study's authors cautioned that the suspected correlation needed more study.

In 2014, the 9th European Breast Cancer Conference was told that sport activities for more than an hour a day would reduce the risk of contracting breast cancer. Those findings, extrapolated from an examination of 37 studies published between 1987 and 2013, represented more than four million women. The results, it was said, applied to women of virtually all ages, weight and geographic locations.

Another recent survey indicated females were reaching puberty at younger ages, as early as 7 or 8. Its results, which looked at 1,239 girls, troubled some observers. They feared the data confirmed earlier studies linking early puberty to higher post-menopausal breast cancer risk.

What else is being put under a microscope?

An associate professor at Dominican University in San Rafael, California, a short crow's flight from my home, reportedly was exploring the potential link in 2012 between chronic cadmium exposure and breast cancer. Cadmium, a heavy metal, as a rule is found in cosmetics, food, water and air particles, rechargeable batteries and cigarette smoke.

One more survey, out of Stanford close to the same time, said researchers working with mice found that a single antibody could shrink or eliminate breast cancer tumors as well as a range of similar growths on the ovaries, prostate, colon, liver, bladder and brain.

Studies on humans had a long way to go, however.

After heavy doses of research, IORT — intra-operative radiation therapy — started to take hold in 2012 as an alternative to longer radiation treatments and more radiation exposure to tissue around a tumor. Other benefits of the treatment, which could be done at the same time as a lumpectomy, were said to be less risk of recurrence, fewer side effects, less pain and fewer skin problems.

And late that year, a story in The New York Times reported that a new genome survey, focused on common classifications believed to originate in the milk duct, had "identified four genetically distinct types" of breast cancer. The expectation was that the study, which concentrated on early, non-metastasized cancers, would "lead to new treatments with drugs already approved for cancers in other parts of the body."

What was needed? Clinical trials, more clinical trials and, yes, still more clinical trials.

What, meanwhile, is *not* needed by patients and caregivers? Disinformation. Or misinformation. But they're both widespread. So is political chicanery.

Consider, for instance, a 2012 Nicholas D. Kristof column in The New York Times titled "The Cancer Lobby," in which he charged the chemical industry has tried to quash a report on carcinogens, "a 500-page consensus document published every two years by the National Institutes of Health."

Kristof's piece also maintained that formaldehyde, which is used in building materials, causing us to breathe its fumes, "is found in everything from nail polish to kitchen countertops, fabric softeners to carpets" and causes cancer of the nose and throat and, possibly, leukemia.

Plain ol' confusion can also cause apprehension among potential breast cancer patients, which translates into all women (and a smattering of men).

A law that went into effect throughout California in 2013 called for doctors to notify women with dense breast tissue (about 40 percent) they could be at a heightened risk for the disease and should check out testing options in addition to mammography (such as a sonogram or MRI).

That, in spite of the lack of a clear-cut definition for dense tissue.

The very definition of the word "cancer," in fact, went under the microscope in in mid-2013 when advisers of the National Cancer Institute suggested it be altered (and softened) — and that the term itself, and variants, be surgically removed from some common diagnoses (such as ductal carcinoma *in situ*).

Why the recommendation? Those experts felt the changes might eliminate the dread some patients experience at the mere mention of the word.

Surprise. Major disagreement erupted in the medical community.

But it seems almost any modern research can trigger controversy —or at least confusion.

A 2012 study found almost half the women who had lumpectomies underwent second operations that might have been unnecessary. Why? Because surgeons were uncertain about guidelines regarding how wide safe-margins should be.

As I was busy perusing facts about that report, the wife of a guy in my Man to Man support group was flying her blood to a German lab that claimed to have found a way to determine which chemo drugs would work on which patients.

Research, of course, takes endless forms and occurs in thousands of places. Monetary support for that research also comes from a vast diversity of sources. Some of them are out of the ordinary.

Such as San Quentin State Prison, where 300 inmates took part in an almost 200-lap prison yard fundraising walk that coincided with a mid-2014 Avon Walk simultaneously taking place in nearby San Francisco.

Regardless whether any of tomorrow's research will actually turn a corner in fighting the disease, one survey commissioned by the Breast Cancer Research Foundation was significantly downbeat. It said 70 percent of U.S. women believe there's been little or no progress in finding a cure. And a second study claimed more than a quarter of the 6,000 people examined thought there was nothing they could do to protect themselves from getting one cancer or another.

As a rule, I'm pleased to say, hopelessness of that sort still can change into hopefulness once a woman recognizes she's not a statistic but an individual.

And hope — the classic needlepoint ceaselessly informs us — springs eternal.

12
AS MORE YEARS GO BY

There's no question my marriage to Nancy has been colored by the post-cancer assurance that the only time we have is now.

Sometimes I've taken charge, sometimes she has.

Sometimes we've stayed on an equal footing — even when tension pushed me into "fight or flight" mode.

Along the way I've learned to lean on whatever grabs my attention, such as an anxiety-allaying 16-page brochure from Y-Me, a Chicago-based national support organization that, unfortunately, folded its tents in mid-2012.

The booklet, "When The Woman You Love Has Breast Cancer," observed that, "contrary to myths, breast cancer is rarely the cause of divorce. Typically, relationships that were strong before the diagnosis of breast cancer remain strong after surgery and treatment."

Its introduction also noted that "the traditional male role — solving problems and acting knowledgeable, protective and in charge — may be causing you turmoil. You may even be experiencing guilt over worrying about your own emotional pain.

"These feelings are normal."

Those four words may be the most important the partner of a breast cancer patient will ever read. With his world turned upside down and inside out, knowing there is a "normal" cannot be over-emphasized.

The pamphlet accurately pointed out your mate "may experience fear, denial, frustration, isolation, confusion, guilt, anxiety and a sense of betrayal. Many women understandably change their everyday priorities, putting themselves first…Your partner may distance herself from you, physically and emotionally, to protect you from potential loss."

Male caregivers, it added, may feel some of the same emotions as the patient, and go through "a variety of emotional and psychosomatic problems."

Sadly, the passing years only underscored the fact that not much information was available to help men straining to give their partners extra help — whether the subject was diet, exercise, fear, perspective, demographics, or the aftermath of breast cancer and its treatments.

Consider the mountains of data on food: women clearly are the prime target; men are, once again, a forgotten part of the equation.

Immediately after her diagnosis, my wife grew uptight about the waist-expanding goodies she was stuffing into her mouth faster than a politician can excuse his screwups.

Eating too much had become a giant societal no-no for healthy living. And most experts lined up behind the notion that proper diets also lead to longevity when coupled with adequate exercise. But dieting suggestions tended to be as ubiquitous, as unreliable and contradictory as wartime press releases from the military.

Newsweek once looked at the big picture in a piece that blamed breast and other cancers on faulty diets. "Poor eating habits," it decreed, "account for a third" of them.

A National Cancer Institute report indicated, around the same time, that breast cancer rates in the United States were four to seven times higher than in Asia. Yet, according to the study, when Asians relocated to the United States, their risk reached ours in several generations.

Why?

Apparently because participants changed their diets, consuming more meat, fat and calories and not eating as many grains, veggies and fruits as they did in their native lands.

While the diet research was being spewed out and challenged, no one seemed to dispute the merits of exercise.

Patients, caregivers and healers paid particular attention when the New England Journal detailed a survey proclaiming exercise could significantly reduce the risk of breast cancer. A total of 25,624 Norwegian women between the ages of 20 and 50 had been tracked for 14 years. Those who exercised regularly reportedly had a 37 percent lower risk of breast cancer than those who didn't.

After reading that, I playfully suggested to Nance, "Women at risk can exercise and establish good diet habits in one fell swoop — by regularly toting home massive crates of veggies."

We did worship at the altar of exercise, though.

As I panted on a treadmill and stationary bike, and my partner adopted dog walking as her main workout, a small group of breast cancer survivors had a much loftier goal — climbing Mount Aconcagua in Argentina to prove the disease couldn't stop them. Three years later, a dozen women tried to scale Mount McKinley, Alaska's tallest peak, but couldn't reach the 20,320-foot summit because of exposure to high winds, below zero and incredibly hot temperatures, whiteouts and a virus that spread through the group.

Nance preferred to "do her own thing" — like climb what she called a "personal mountain" in Beijing. So she and I trudged up 1,180 uneven steps of the Great Wall of China, a brick-and-mortar, man-made miracle extending more than 4,000 miles around a comparatively small part of the country's perimeter.

The heat slowed our pace. Sweat drenched us both.

Every few hundred stairs, as we'd hit yet one more outlook point, I asked, "Isn't this sufficient. How many more steps do you need to climb?"

"I'll let you know when we're high enough," my wife would say, her smile as wide as the smog-covered vistas.

When we reached what she arbitrarily decided was "our pinnacle," having outlasted virtually every other tourist, and stepping higher than our Chinese guide had climbed before, Nance and I gave each other a high-five, pumped our arms in victory and shouted "Yes!"

She later called the feat "a triple joy."

"First," she said, "was my ability, at age 59, to do it."

Because it was her moment of triumph, I stayed politely silent about being two years her senior and 70 pounds heavier. But, almost as if she'd heard my unspoken thought, she announced to the thinned air her second bit of delight — "an appreciation, once again, of my husband, my partner, who moved upward today with me, by my side despite his own discomfort, knowing this ascent was important to me."

Then she detailed her third, and top, priority — "getting there to celebrate being alive, vital and a survivor of breast cancer."

On the way up, as we periodically stopped to feel grateful how far we'd traveled, other significant life-steps trickled into our consciousness: the cancer tests, the lumpectomy, the infusion of poison chemicals into Nance's veins, the radiation treatments, the visualizations, the support groups, the ingestion of myriad vitamins, and the endless tears and laughs.

At the peak, we reveled in our success. We had earned the matching "I climbed the Great Wall of China" T-shirts we would later buy far below.

But no vendor among the thousands and thousands in Beijing had created the shirts we really wanted:

"We climbed the Great Wall — of Cancer."

Scrambling up heights, even with a partner or in a group, is always an individual achievement. So is facing the end of life.

We attended a friend's funeral in San Francisco. Her breast cancer had returned after an absence of 16 years. It instantly slammed the nightmare into our faces again.

It reminded us that when Nance's cancer hit it tore away all the safety nets we thought we had. At the time, she hid from me what she'd written; it was too raw, she believed. *"I do know that I'm scared out of my wits. It's the kind of fear that makes your blood run cold, the sort of fear that floods in when you lose sight of your child in a crowd."*

She certainly wasn't the only frightened person in cancer's anteroom.

I can't count how often I started to quarrel with her over something insignificant because I needed to vent my anxiety or anger at her being sick but couldn't.

Nor can I count how often I wanted to flee from our wedlock, fueled by a hundred minor irritants or a fear attack.

My biggest apprehension? That Nance's breast cancer would return and kill her.

My second largest? That my courage quotient wouldn't equal hers.

Not long after her treatments ended, Nance said, "I realize, and I guess all of us realize, in effect there are *no* cancer survivors, that we all must live with cancer all the time."

She was right, of course, but neither she nor I wanted to accept that "all the time" truly meant *all the time.*

Time itself had become problematic for us.

Like so many other basic elements of our lives, it depended on the way we perceived it. Slow. Slower. Stop. Fast. Faster. Rush. It also depended on what we stirred into the mix. Cancer can rearrange one's outlook faster than a bullet train in Japanese mountains.

Many spiritual leaders like to turn the disease on its head and label it "a gift." They say its life-threatening qualities put things in "true perspective."

Mostly, we find that accurate if a bit hard to swallow.

Trivial things that once disturbed us faded into the background as soon as Nancy was diagnosed. Doing a load of wash could wait. So could dozens of daily chores that once upon a time seemed crucial. So, in fact, could our occupations, and my writing.

My wife became my biggest champion, though. She urged me to finish the manuscript for this book, and to include as many paragraphs of humor as possible. We agreed laughter is one of the best unguents for breast cancer.

Yes, but while humor can definitely ease stress, anxiety can be malignant.

Witness the night terrors about my mortality that detonated when a lump the size of a ping-pong ball grew on my tongue.

My wife clutched my hand as the pathologist conducted a biopsy in his office-lab. "I can't separate the pain your grip is causing me from the anxiety due to the thing in my mouth," I said.

Nance said nothing.

"I didn't want him to have cancer," she later wrote in her journal.

"The thought that his tongue could be damaged, his speech impaired, his job threatened, his communication with the rest of the world made difficult, and, most importantly, his life put on the line, scared me."

When we got home, Nance guided me through a visualization exercise:

"I'm on a Caribbean shoreline, in a beach chair, sipping a cool drink through a straw," I told her, my eyes shut tightly. "Hovering over me is Superman, my boyhood superhero, cape and all.

"I pay no attention to the fact that he's a comic-book character. He's humanoid, and he's there for me.

"He pops the cyst on my tongue. It explodes into thousands of tiny fragments. The particles flutter to the ground, burying themselves in the white sand. My tongue heals by itself, without medication or surgery or any more help from Superman. I smile."

When I opened my eyes, I was still smiling.

For the next few days, though, neither Nance nor I slept well — waiting several days for test results was hellfire like no other.

The doctor got to Nance first because he couldn't reach me. My lump was not malignant.

"The relief I experienced was unbelievable," she wrote. *"I was thrilled. I sighed. I yelled. I couldn't wait to tell Woody when I saw him, since he was already commuting home. It was a delicious moment when I blurted out the good news."*

We agreed, when the growth disappeared on its own a few weeks later, to turn the episode — and our pointless worry — into our 4,219th medical anecdote.

It may have been a little off the wall but we were overjoyed to return to thinking about my wife and her no-longer-present breast cancer. Once again we could see that an affirmative perspective is crucial.

Without question, Nance had lucked out.

She wasn't poor. Or black.

A study looking into why fewer African-American women survived breast cancer than white females found that poor women were less likely to be diagnosed. Consequently, they were less apt to be treated for the disease and, therefore, more prone to die from it.

A 2012 Washington Post series said the toll among black females stemmed in large part from fear and a lack of information. A July 2013 column in The New York Times cited a study containing some horrifying statistics, including the fact that "black patients are twice as likely to never receive treatment."

The column also indicated that "white women with breast cancer lived three years longer than black women," and that, "of the women studied, nearly 70 percent of white women lived at least five years after diagnosis, while 56 percent of black women were alive five years later."

Only 23.5 percent of black women, it reported, had been screened for breast cancer "six to eighteen months before diagnosis, compared with 35.7 percent of white women."

A Times article in 2013 underscored those findings. It noted that Memphis is the "deadliest major American city for African-American women with breast cancer" — with twice as many there likely to die of the disease than whites. It indicated, too, that starting in the 1990s, advances in care became widely available in early detection and treatment throughout the country — for Caucasians but not for blacks.

The American Cancer Society earlier had reported cancer patients with no health insurance — who accordingly were less liable to get screening tests — were twice as likely to die within five years as those with private coverage.

Without question, Nance had lucked out. She wasn't a pariah.

Appallingly, society too often treated cancer patients — and, of course, persons with AIDS — like the lepers of yesteryear.

The Associated Press reported cancer patients nationally being fired or laid off five times as often as other people. One in 14 were victimized in that way. And when patients kept their jobs, a study showed, they often were stripped of important duties by supervisors.

The results came from a survey, issued by Working Woman magazine, which included interviews with 100 supervisors, 100 co-workers and 500 cancer survivors who remained on the job while in treatment. It showed 85 percent of supervisors believed cancer survivors working for them suffered fatigue while undergoing chemo; only 58 percent of patients actually did. Nausea was cited by 74 percent of the supervisors, though only 33 percent of the diseased had that side effect.

Without question, I had lucked out, too.

I managed to find the inner resources to overcome my sense that caregiving is similar to parachuting from a plane and not finding a ripcord.

From time to time, though, I'd still find myself fretting that breast cancer cost me a robust sex life. The lack of post-cancer sexual intercourse can scramble to the top of the side-effects chart — behind hair loss for women, I guess, but numero uno for loads of male caregivers.

The medical community plays down the loss of sexual appetite, focusing instead on the cancer itself. But when the immediate danger wanes, patients and partners can't ignore the changes that chemo fashions.

Nance long had been aware I was displeased with her inattention. But she tried to laugh it off as just another manifestation of "chemo-brain," a term she and others in her group typically applied to forgetfulness.

Eventually we decided to see a psychologist together. Nance had wept as she told him of her exasperation at not being able to satisfy me. "I want to," she said, "but it hurts."

The therapist could only suggest what we already knew: Sexual activity needn't be limited to vaginal intercourse.

Our acceptance occurred only after Nance's gynecologist told us that my wife, mainly because of the chemo, had "a shortened vagina with thin walls that are hyper-sensitive."

The doc would figuratively give intercourse "last rites" and advise, only half in jest, that I try a blowup doll.

Had physicians warned up front that sexual activity might be severely curtailed, I'd probably have said, "Okay, it's a fair trade — intercourse for her life." But their total silence about the subject ultimately angered me.

The female side of it had been addressed in a New York City symposium titled "Sex After Breast Cancer." All four panelists agreed when a woman underwent a mastectomy and chemo, more than the physical was lost. "Feelings of worthlessness, and a decline in a sense of attractiveness" are among those losses, said one psychology professor.

Similar reactions, the panelists unanimously iterated, could be expected from women who'd had lumpectomies.

"Sex is a symbol in our society, a measure of social worth, mental health, love and intimacy," said a second psych prof. "Cancer often requires the couple to redesign their way of intimately relating to each other."

While Nance and I were learning to deal with our intimacy problem, marketing experts struggled with the general public's collective mind-set on breast cancer. Because of a growing outcry about the disease — predominantly from women voters — Congress had approved legislation authorizing the sale of a special "semi-postal stamp," the first in history, to raise research money.

The initial attempt unfortunately became a public relations debacle.

Bureaucratic glitches and logistical difficulties took their toll: Approval was given for the stamp's face value to be the same as regular issues. The stamp might evoke awareness of the disease, but there would be no proceeds to fight it.

To say breast cancer warriors were upset is like saying General Custer was slightly miffed at Little Big Horn.

A second try worked better, though it took two years to straighten things out.

A breast cancer stamp featuring a mythological Roman goddess ultimately was minted. It showed Diana pulling an arrow from a quiver. Her right arm, raised behind her head, was positioned for breast self-exam. Encircling her right breast was the slogan "Fund the fight. Find a cure."

It came to pass after a survey showed consumers willing to buy stamps eight cents higher than normal.

The premium was earmarked for the National Institutes of Health (70 percent) and the medical research program of the Department of Defense (30 percent).

Before you could shout pop culture, the stamp became a bestseller, knocking the Bugs Bunny design out of second place. Only the Elvis issue had more sales. The breast cancer stamp would raise tens of millions of dollars for research and, along with awareness month, bolster the disease's visibility.

Breast cancer, it quickly become apparent, was on a fast track to becoming a populist ailment.

People magazine had featured the subject as early as 1998. Its celebrity cover story, titled "Surviving Breast Cancer," spotlighted photos of, among others, Shirley Temple Black, Gloria Steinem, Julia Child and Peggy Fleming.

The awareness bandwagon had its own side effect for Nance and me: It would help us stay balanced. Every cheerleading paragraph would become a panel in our metaphoric healing quilt — as would each incident that taught us a new lesson.

One day a heavy metal door slammed behind us, trapping us in a San Francisco stairwell. We pounded on the rear entryways to several commercial shops.

No one heard.

As we discussed what to do next, a door to a Chinese restaurant opened. An employee wearing a grease-splattered apron came out to sneak a cigarette. He spoke no English. We walked by him into the bowels of the restaurant. As we strutted past the wide-eyed staff, I said to my partner, "There's a good message here. Even when we think we're trapped, if we're patient, a way out of a difficult spot will appear."

Nance and I relished that we had the knack, like modern alchemists, of changing bothersome events into our personal bumper stickers.

We also appreciated that, as her after-care progressed, media outlets had been running more and more tales about the breast cancer epidemic and how people could deal with it.

The San Francisco Chronicle, for example, had published one about 40 men and women who acted as a surrogate family for a co-worker. They'd shopped for her, cooked her meals, drove her to medical appointments and, toward the end, stayed with her round the clock.

A sidebar offered tips on how to aid workmates facing life-threatening diseases, including:

- Taking your cues from the ill worker ("Some people want a lot of support; others prefer to handle their illnesses privately").
- Feeling free "to offer health information…but don't shove your personal advice or 'cure' down his or her throat."
- Helping in concrete ways, such as doing errands or laundry — not pressuring the sick person to be cheerful ("Comments like 'You're so brave' can make people feel obligated to put on a facade of happiness").
- Remembering the caregivers ("taking care of a sick partner, child or parent can be as draining as the illness itself").

My wife and I deemd the dissemination of tips like those promising. And we looked upon fundraisers for research as another positive.

When Nance collected money as part of her participation in the Race for the Cure, the biggest donation she received was $500. But it was the smallest that had gotten to me.

A Russian émigre working at a foundation she consulted for came up to her with a crumpled one-dollar bill.

"I'm poor," she said. "This is all I can afford but I want to support what you're doing."

How many dollars and how many mouse and human lifetimes will it take breast cancer researchers to find a cure?

In 1971, President Richard Nixon had signed into law the National Cancer Act, a couple of years after he "declared war" on the disease.

One payoff from the attention garnered by the funding law was an over-all drop in the death rate for the first time.

That fact moved the National Cancer Institute's director to strut like a peacock. "This," predicted Dr. Richard Klausner, "is the news we've been waiting for. The 1990s will be remembered as the decade when we measurably turned the tide against cancer."

Another more current improvement on the breast cancer front came in the form of node surgery.

A new technique let surgeons pinpoint the first pea-sized node under the arm likely to turn malignant. Physicians then could remove that node alone. If that turned out to be benign, the rest could be spared (at least for early breast cancer patients).

A study released in 2011 underscored earlier findings that showed removal of a sentinel node as accurate a predictor as cutting them all out. The discovery overturned a 100-year-old medical practice.

It would arrive too late, of course, to benefit Nance or thousands of others.

But after years and years on the front lines of the breast cancer war, she and I were thrilled to report we felt life would go on.

She wrote in her diary:

"I find myself saying, to myself and to others, when things go 'wrong,' 'This should be the worst thing that ever happens to you.' That doesn't mean I don't get bothered, irritated or annoyed. It just means I have a different set of lenses through which I view them.

"The cancer's made me conscious of my frailty as a human being, conscious that each day is a gift — something I knew but not the way I know now. I'm aware cancer could recur at any second, but I don't live in fear that it will. My energy is focused instead on staying healthy.

"I want us all to be healthy and to stay that way. Healthy of body, spirit and mind. So I can write some more about this in another five years. And five years after that, and after that, and after that."

From her mouth to God's heart.

13
TWENTY YEARS LATER

The crummy news is, not every breast cancer patient has survived, and not every researcher has made progress in the early 21st century. And some items fit the aphorism "the more things change, the more they stay the same."

Way back in 1993, The New York Times Magazine had run a cover photo of a woman with her chest bared, her breast cancer scar visible. It caused a public stir and a private debate among journalists as to whether the picture was appropriate. Discussions faded without resolution.

Almost a decade later, a similar debate hit several communities in the Bay Area.

Controversial billboard and poster ads, part of a Breast Cancer Fund awareness campaign, became the center of political skirmishes. Some of the ads showed models with single mastectomies. And one portrayed a bare-chested woman in a sexy pose — one hand on a rounded hip, another on a thigh. Her lips were pursed. But her breasts were missing, replaced by scars.

All the computer-enhanced advertisements were banned in San Francisco, a city known for sexually explicit Halloween block parties and gay-pride parades, not to mention nude marchers during its annual Bay-to-Breakers foot races.

The head of the ad agency holding exclusive rights to bus-shelter advertising in the city simply found the photos too rough. "To see a woman's terribly, terribly scarred body — it's just not for public consumption on the streets of San Francisco...where children and others can be traumatized," he said. "It's too shocking. Too upsetting. Too provocative."

The controversy died a natural death so no one uttered a word for years about photos of breast-less women being more offensive than, let's say, coffins bearing dead U.S. warriors from Afghanistan.

During the 20 years following Nance's diagnosis, thankfully, there have been many advances in regard to breast cancer — and many other diseases, including the prostate cancer I contracted.

But breasts remain contentious.

In 2011, several American school districts banned wristbands and T-shirts that said "I [heart] Boobies," and in October of that year, cheerleaders at an Arizona high school were barred from wearing pink T-shirts with the slogan "Feel for lumps, save your bumps."

Inappropriate, said administrators, ignoring the teens' goal of raising funds for breast cancer research.

In 2013, a U.S. Court of Appeals ruled in a 9-5 decision that school districts can't ban bracelets with "boobies" slogans. But Pennsylvania's Eaton School District later voted to appeal the ruling.

Will the free-speech issue end up in the lap of Supreme Court justices? Only God and a bevy of attorneys know.

That same year, The New York Times was the center of a political firestorm once again, this time in print magazines, online and especially on Twitter — because it ran a Page One photo showing part of an areola along with a lumpectomy scar. Critics claimed the article about breast cancer gene testing in Israel objectified women and sexualized both the breast and the cancer; defenders labeled the criticism misogynistic claptrap.

And in 2014, the Huffington Post reported a major flap caused by a British ad proclaiming "I Wish I Had Breast Cancer."

Pancreatic Cancer Action had placed the advertisement with the intent of showing how lethal that disease is compared to other common cancers. Objectors — including friends of ours who firmly believe getting a life-threatening disease may be a gift from God so recipients and caregivers can fully appreciate each day — called it outrageous (and added a few obscenities).

While those furors were getting scads of attention, non-sensational accounts about breast cancer and related topics typically were relegated to the back of surviving newspapers.

Or cut to three-paragraph shorts.

It could be hard, for example, to find in-depth pieces in print or online about chemo-brain — the woolly-headedness that cancer patients gripe about during treatment — despite research showing that the condition can last as long as a patient lives.

Findings from a Dartmouth Medical School study nonetheless warned ordinary doses of chemo might permanently dull survivors' brainpower, resulting in bad memories, muddy thinking, an inability to do mathematical calculations mentally, and a need to read a page twice to absorb its content.

Not that long ago, I found another breast cancer story buried in the rear sections of several papers.

The Associated Press dispatch, which definitely rattled me, said elderly spouses "strained by caring for an ailing husband or wife were 63 percent more likely to die than other spouses."

They succumbed to heart disease, stroke, cancer, pneumonia and kidney failure.

Frankly, I prefer not to dwell on the nugatory, not on the stress of being a healing partner, but rather on the feel-good moments of my life — and how much good advice we've been given since Nancy's diagnosis.

Among the best came from a Kaiser Permanente Medical Center breast-care coordinator, Mary Beth Faustine, during my wife's treatments: "Don't make radical lifestyle alterations, like adopting a rigorous diet or changing your religion."

That tip worked so well because my wife and I both needed ways to stay grounded. We'd felt there was no safe place, that we'd been thrust into a lightning storm with tall metal poles taped to our hands.

"It's clear," I said at one point, "that from now on we've got to be ready to change on a second's notice, to adjust to whatever the 'new normal' is. And we'll probably have to do it repeatedly without ever being able to properly weigh the evidence."

I grinned. "Outside of that, of course, everything will remain exactly the way it always was."

Some revisions Nance had to make were minor (yet of great magnitude to her). After months of post-treatment hunting in women's boutique shops and department stores, for instance, she'd found a wireless bra that fit perfectly and didn't hurt where the surgery had taken place.

As each year passed, like an insect drawn to a torn packet of sugar, I learned to perform whatever mental or spiritual heavy lifting was necessary. To wit:

- I enjoyed twisting a cynical bumper sticker into, "Life may be a bitch, but then you live."
- When I was diagnosed with diabetes, my first reaction was depression, but then, "It's okay — it's not cancer." Years later, during a single week, a flu bug drained me, cracks disfigured

our deck, the cable TV quit, a favorite sweater tore at the neckline, our computer croaked, my wipers stopped in mid-thunderstorm, and Nance's rental house was gutted in a fire. Oh, yeah, I split my trousers on the way to work. But, as I told my wife, "I don't have cancer, and neither do you."

- I found it impossible not to appreciate a higher power's hands in our journey.

I learned, too, to *really* hear what others had to teach. Witness the words of one of Nance's support group members on an anniversary of their first meeting:

"When diagnosed, I was afraid I would die young...After surviving breast cancer, I felt I could survive almost anything. My fear of flying disappeared; I demolished my car and was unaffected by it. I love life, and my motto is, 'You live until you die,' so I try to live daily with a positive attitude."

That perspective's easy for me to believe *now*, 20 years out. Obviously it wasn't always that way.

Nance and I occasionally relive our bumpy breast cancer coaster ride. We'll certainly never forget the grueling months of surgery, radiation and chemotherapy.

But we've also learned how to count our blessings — even when I was struck with prostate cancer.

What girded me for that cancer?

Topping the list, in addition to my father's losing bout with the disease: Nancy's breast cancer and melanoma and our subsequent years crammed with evocative, remarkable lessons.

I learned, as the main byproduct of being a caregiving partner, to glean something upbeat from each day. I internalized what some might find slightly mawkish but totally worked for me, the notion that if today feels like a cloudy mess, tomorrow will almost certainly outshine it.

I still had to quash my demons.

Toward the end of my treatments I wrote an e-mail that said: "I knew I was getting better when I was able to kvetch...about my right shoulder hurting from arthritis...and about the sundry discolorations on my body that keep it from being a perfect specimen (snickering is definitely appropriate)."

Not exactly stellar material for a stand-up.

Yes, trying to unearth a pebble's worth of humor from a quarry of adversity is sometimes a stretch.

I also reached out to a God I wasn't sure existed. In an extremely reflective column I noted that my final treatment, an in-patient surgical procedure, had left me, a self-styled control freak, with "no control whatsoever" — and that "the San Francisco operating room had unexpectedly become my foxhole, the clichéd place where there are no atheists or agnostics."

Over and over and over again, I wrote, "silent words" engulfed my brain: *"Thank you God, for healing me. Thank you God, for extending my life. Thank you God. Thank you."*

After treatment upon treatment and what the U.S. Supreme Court once termed "deliberate speed," my liberator, my knight in white armor — a brand new "new normal" — eventually materialized.

And I was okay.

At one point I'd sent an e-mail message to Man to Man regulars that cited my gratitude for "the opportunity to bitch about my hormonal and radiation side effects. I'm alternating hot flashes and cold flashes, I'm having night sweats, I'm weeping in the middle of conversations, I'm cranky, I'm belching and farting, and my bowels are in a semi-constant proverbial uproar. But each side effect is simply proof that the treatments are killing the cancer."

When tests showed I was cancer-free and apt to stay that way, Nance and I reviewed the impact our respective diseases had had on us — as well as a few tips we'd picked up along the way that we might share with others.

- We suggest finding a support group pronto (if the first or second isn't to your liking, try another).
- We recommend downloading or renting comedies, taking nature walks and reading or listening to whatever brings you pleasure.
- We urge patients to encircle themselves with peers who can evoke positive feelings or laughter.
- And, lastly, we encourage patients to do whatever they've postponed for a lifetime (whatever's possible today, without waiting until tomorrow or the day after).

We normally ask those we counsel to look at the fact that both Nance and I have conquered our cancers, as have millions of others, and to recognize we're still here, extraordinarily alive and definitively kicking.

Getting through any life-threatening disease admittedly can be likened to inching through an amusement park's sinister House of Horrors. But once a sightseer is back in the sunlight, smiling can become almost effortless. A personal memory may illustrate the point:

Nance's mammogram showed a spot in 2009. Scary enough, in fact, to bring her to tears. A second mammogram showed it "was nothing." And that, of course, brought relief.

But the old fears and horrific memories had surfaced again.

She experienced yet another nerve-wracking blip in 2010. A routine visit to her gynecologist uncovered a new lump on her right breast, the one that had had the cancer. The doctor said it most likely was just a cyst but suggested we see a specialist to be sure.

A week later Nance was given a mammogram, a sonogram and a touchy-feely exam by a surgeon. The composite verdict: A non-malignant, non-problematic oily cyst. We hustled back to relief land.

Breathing can become such a luxury.

I much prefer relying on more positive recollections.

A friend who'd been a professional clown for years had e-mailed us after a bout with breast cancer and treatments that left nerve damage. "I feel so blessed," she'd written in a bi-level punch-line, "to still being able to make a fool of myself."

Some outsiders might suspect that with prostate cancer and diabetes, as well as the stress of dealing with both of Nance's cancers, I'd be falling apart. But they'd be wrong.

I continued to focus on survival.

So I was particularly pleased in 2012 when the Man to Man group expanded its horizons by having our first male breast cancer survivor join us as a regular.

Then we expanded even further: A guy whose wife had lung cancer found we could help him cope.

In 2014, my 48-year-old son fell at work, fracturing his hip. A surgical replacement was required. I flew to Atlanta, where he lived alone, to ease his recovery. The month-long visit became an instant refresher course in caregiving, a booster shot that flashed me back to being on call 24/7 during Nance's breast cancer treatments and aftermath, as well as during her recovery from foot surgery years later.

Because both she and I had survived our personal rollercoasters, the memories were almost wholly constructive.

The truth is, not even the economic downturn could shake us.

We realized, of course, that our narrative might benefit anyone who faces — with a caregiving partner or alone — cancer of whatever kind, AIDS or, indeed, any life-threatening disease.

Especially pertinent, we believed, is that each of our crises had brought us closer together.

Yes, there are times even now when I'm less than the perfect partner — when I'm totally selfish or when I growl or yell at my wife. But I've never felt so whole.

I remain mindful of my body (having revamped my diet), my mind (making sure it stays active) and, above all, my spirit (I intend to keep filling my life with every possible goody until my last breath).

The truth is, I'm counting on my wife and me dying together in a plane crash in Tibet or some totally unreachable place when I'm 96 and she's only 94.

Unless it happens later.

14
AFTERWORD

During our wedding ceremony, Nancy recited these words to me:

"Is that you, Woody, with your infinite eyes, deep and loving, just as they were then, in the snow?

"Is that you, Woody, with those self-same eyes peeking now over grandpa glasses perched on the tip of your nose?

"Is that you, Woody, with your thunderous laughter, amazed by my six-year-old clown and my 'cast of thousands'?

"Is that you, Woody, with your critical eye, inspiring my muses, encouraging my truth?

"Is that you, Woody, right in the ring with me, making me the best me I can be?

"Is that you, Woody, being my mother and father, sister and brother, grandma and grandpa, cousins, lover, and friend?

"Is that you, Woody, changing, and changed, changer and changee?

"Yup, that's you, Woody!

"And this is me, in middle-age-woman makeup, standing beside you today just to tell you I love you, and I'll be your wife.

"There, I said the 'w' word."

Nance's humor and lightness, as always, camouflaged apprehensions and doubts. Just before the ceremony she'd told a friend she was nervous about jumping with me "into a merger-matic."

It took years, and a sprinkling of therapy, for the "w" word to fit comfortably. Then, abruptly leaping from the shadows, the "c" word had kidnapped us, turning my wife into a breast cancer patient and me into a caregiver, stuffing us both into a single rollercoaster seat.

It's been a long and often scary trip, significantly more protracted and difficult than anticipated. Even today, passing the 20-year mark, we'd joyfully trade in all we've learned, all the affection propelled in our direction, for a guarantee no cancer will recur.

We know, however, there can be no assurances, and that we are permanently changed.

We can now offer greater understanding and kindness to each other — and to virtually everyone who touches our lives. We can now recognize it's not crucial what gender or age someone with a life-threatening disease is, and that both designated patient and anointed caregiver require nurturing.

We can more regularly keep our priorities in order, strive for balance, unblock our spirituality and divert the million potential intrusions on our lives each week.

The day we wed, I read these vows to my wife-to-be:

"I knew you, lifetimes ago, as Nancy Falk, a cute freckle-faced teenager, with bright jade eyes and an innocent freshness possible only in those from the unspoiled Midwest.

"I know you, now, as Nancy Fox, a lovely freckle-faced child-woman of middle years, with bright jade eyes and a rainbowed mind possible only in those who have tasted the flavors of life's pains and pleasures.

"I will know you, through multiple tomorrows, as Nance, my wife, an elegant freckle-faced woman of timeless beauty, with bright jade eyes and an evolved soul possible only in those whose hearts have opened as exquisitely as a matured rose.

"Through all the nows and yet-to-comes, I pledge only this: to love you without reservation, as fully as the human condition will allow; to nurture our creative talents, so our individual and collective light may brighten a few shadowy corners of this dimension; and to cherish and retain, always, my glorious vision of us as soulmates, a clairvoyant insight reflecting the majesty of our spirits, our highest selves in perfect union."

Love, we've told each other again and again during this ordeal, recovery and aftermath, is the key to all healing. No matter what else science has figured out, it still hasn't determined how to put that into a test tube and measure it.

Although Nance's breast cancer treatments activated a torrent of disagreeable side effects, they simultaneously fortified our adoration for each other. As a result of the illness, and despite occasionally waking with formless terror, we've re-vowed to love and support each other the way we believe soulmates must.

For decades to come.

Every now and then we pause to deal with some reminder of what we've weathered, what we've survived.

On the 19th anniversary of her diagnosis, for instance, we shredded documents about Nance's cancer that filled several cardboard boxes we'd been storing out of sight.

On the 20th anniversary, we traveled to Paris and London as a well-earned celebration.

For now, we're consumed once again — not by breast cancer or a melanoma or prostate cancer this time, not by thoughts of physical or mental anguish, but by a bright horizon as seen from the crest of the rollercoaster.

Each day, each month, each year gets better and better. We get closer and closer. Our lives are wrapped in more and more colors, with more texture.

Death eventually will snag us both. But instead of waiting, we're re-experiencing our fairy tale.

One day at a time.

And once again, we've gotten the hang of living happily ever after.

THE END

15
WHERE MEN CAN FIND HELP

Male partners of breast cancer patients may discover someone — or something — to which they can relate in this list of paperback and hardcover books (many of which can be purchased, used, for pennies online). Some also can be found in e-book versions that can be downloaded inexpensively.

- "Breast Cancer Husband: How to Help Your Wife (and Yourself) Through Diagnosis, Treatment and Beyond," by Marc Silver. 304 pages. Rodale. 2004. Paperback. $15.95. Lengthy volume contains lots of information, but has annoying format with small sidebars that interrupt the main flow, plus chapter-ending tips like in a school text.
- "Breast Cancer: Strategies for Husbands to Support Their Wives," by Jim Eckmann. 103 pages. Nehemiah Publishing. 1995. Paperback. $9.95. Thin book, by an author who's published other faith-based volumes, may best help those immersed in Christianity.
- "Confronting the Cow: A Young Family's Struggle with Breast Cancer, Loss and Rebuilding," by C. B. Donner. 240 pages. $21.95. Moonlight Publishing, 2000. A husband and father of four illustrates struggles with his wife dying at age 36.
- "Diary of a Breast Cancer Husband," by J. Scott Lyman. 320 pages. $19.95. Paperback. Times Publishing Group, 2002. A negligence attorney takes a difficult look at his wife's disease and treatment.

- "Helping Your Mate Face Breast Cancer: Tips for Becoming an Effective Support Partner for the One You Love During the Breast Cancer Experience," by Judy C. Kneece. 136 pages. $14.95. Paperback. EduCare Publishing. 1995. Lean volume features interviews, from female perspective, with patients and family members. The author's day-job: oncology nurse.
- "It Takes a Worried Man," by Brendan Halpin. 256 pages. $21.95. Random House, 2002. Riddled with excessive vulgarity, this is a log by a 33-year-old whose wife faces death. The writer seems distant from his mate's plight (except in relation to his pain).
- "Lessons from Joan: Living and Loving with Cancer, A Husband's Story," by Eric R. Kingson. 210 pages. Paperback. $19.95. Syracuse University Press, 2005. This memoir/love story by a professor of social work includes positive messages that may be overshadowed by the death of the woman it depicts.
- "Man to Man: When the Woman You Love Has Breast Cancer," by Andy Murcia and Bob Stewart. 220 pages. Paperback. $16.95. St. Martin's Press, 1989. The main appeal of this book, like a yellowed gossip column, is Murcia's spotlighting the health problems of his actress-celebrity wife, Ann Jillian.
- "Stand By Her: A Breast Cancer Guide for Men," by John W. Anderson. 257 pages. Paperback. $18.95. Amacom/American Management Association, 2009. Writer, from an unusual vantage point of having been surrounded by breast cancer, describes minefields he went through helping his mom, wife, sister and mother's best friend, all of whom had the disease.
- "Survivor's Guide to Breast Cancer: A Couple's Story of Faith, Hope & Love," by Robert C. Fore, Rorie E. Fore and Nancy W. Dickey. 128 pages. Paperback. $17. Smyth & Helwys, 1998. This skinny book, which focuses on divine healing, straddles the views of its husband and wife authors, health-care pros who talk much about the docs and nurses who were their friends.
- "What's the Next Step?" by Robert Fritz. 168 pages. $25.95. iUniverse, 2012. Employing a workbook format, the writer tells of caregiving for his first wife, who died after a 13-year breast cancer battle, and then himself when he contracted brain cancer.
- "When Life Becomes Precious: The Essential Guide for Patients, Loved Ones, and Friends of Those Facing Serious Illnesses," by Elise NeeDell Babcock. 304 pages. Paperback. $16.95. Bantam, 1997. Though not specifically aimed at men, this volume is one

of the best guides available for "those facing serious illnesses," be they caregivers or patients.

- "When the Woman You Love Has Breast Cancer," by Larry T. Eiler. 66 pages. Paperback. $13.95. Queen Bee Publishing, 1994. Slim book, based on personal experience, offers ways to be supportive.
- "When Your Wife Has Breast Cancer: A Story of Love, Courage & Survival," By Mark S. Weiss. 157 pages. $17.95. Brick Tower Press, 2006. A real estate exec, the writer details his initial rigidity and tells how he dealt with despair and frustration.

Not quite what you're looking for? Perhaps these additional resources for male caregivers can lead to good advice or solace.

- **HealthCentral.com.** Segment of broader website — www.MyBreastCancerNetwork.com — is devoted to breast cancer partners and husbands.(703) 302-1040.www.healthcentral.com.
- **Men Against Breast Cancer.** Focuses on how breast cancer affects the family. Provides support and education services. (866) 547-6222. www.menagainstbreastcancer.org.
- **Well Spouse Association.** Gives support to husbands, wives and partners of chronically ill. (800) 838-0879. www.wellspouse.org.
- "Your Partner Has Breast Cancer: 21 Ways to Keep Sane as a Support Person on Your Journey from Victim to Survivor," by Ken Wachsberger. 28-page paperback booklet. $5.50. Azenphony Press, 2001. Brief but to-the-point advice.

Finally, general resources about breast and other cancers include:

- **AMC Cancer Research Center.** Provides information, and has counseling line. (800) 321-1557. www.amc.org.
- **American Cancer Society.** Hotline provides information on all forms of cancer and treatments, and referrals to local support groups, resources and programs. ACS also furnishes brochures and educational materials. And it sponsors Cancer Survivors Network, a web-based service that deals with fears, finances and long-term effects of treatment. (800) 227-2345. www.cancer.org. or www.cancersurvivorsnetwork.org.
- **American Institute for Cancer Research.** Supplies publications and videos on nutrition. (800) 843-8114. www.aicr.org.
- **BreastCancer.org.** Imparts medical information about the disease. (610) 642-6550. www.breastcancer.org.

- **Breast Cancer Alliance.** Presents education and research as part of its overall goal to improve survival rates and quality of life for those impacted by the disease — and proffers support and screening for the uninsured and underserved. (203) 861-0014. www.breastcanceralliance.org.
- **Breast Cancer Care.** London-based clearinghouse for information. Has about 100,000 members in more than 65 online forums discussing thousands of topics. www.breastcancercare.org.uk.
- **Breast Cancer Research Foundation.** Tenders information relating to the disease, heightens awareness of good breast health, and funds research at medical centers worldwide. (646) 497-2600. www.bcrfcure.org.
- **Breast Health Access For Women With Disabilities.** Submits services and education aimed at increasing access and utilization of breast screening by women with limitations in mobility and vision. (510) 204-4574. www.bhawd.org.
- **Canadian Cancer Society.** Offers information, in English and French, from medically approved and complementary therapies, about programs and services in Canada. (306) 566-5700 outside Canada. www.cancer.ca.
- **Cancer Care, Inc.** Presents — for cancer patients and their families — support, education, information, referrals and financial assistance through a counseling line, brochures and a newsletter. (800) 813-4673. www.cancercare.org.
- **Cancer Club.** Provides humorous and helpful books, cassettes and a newsletter. (952) 944-0639. www.cancerclub.com.
- **Cancer Hope Network.** Matches patients and volunteers, and gives counseling about chemotherapy and radiation. (800) 552-4366. www.cancerhopenetwork.org.
- **Cancer Research Institute.** Supplies resource information, and supports research aimed at prevention, treatment and cure. (800) 992-2623. www.cancerresearch.org.
- **Dana Farber Cancer Institute.** Risk line dedicates itself to information about familial cancers. (866) 408-3324. www.dana-farber.org.
- "Dr. Susan Love's Breast Book," by Susan Love, M.D. 736 pages. $22. Paperback. Da Capo Press, fifth edition, 2010. This is the reference bible for breast cancer. www.susanlovemd.com.

- **FORCE,** Facing Our Risk of Cancer Enpowered. Supplies information and support for high-risk women. (866) 288-7475. www.facingourrisk.org.
- **Living Beyond Breast Cancer.** Hotline, staffed by survivors at (888) 753-5222, and organization itself address post-treatment needs through educational programs, newsletter and helpline. Hosts group and programs for young women's needs. (484) 708-1550 or (610) 645-4567. www.lbbc.org.
- **National Breast Cancer Coalition.** Advocates nationally and locally to support legislation and funding that benefits breast cancer patients, survivors and women at risk. (800) 622-2838. www.natlbcc.org.
- **National Breast Cancer Foundation, Inc.** In hopes of saving lives through early detection, supplies free mammograms and breast cancer education (in part via its www.breastcancer.net program, and with the help of a fundraising partner, www.thebreastcancersite.com). (972) 248-9200. www.nationalbreastcancer.org.
- **National Cancer Institute.** Furnishes via print, phone, web and Cancer Information Service network materials on resources, treatments, clinical trials and research. Cancer Information Service: (800) 422-6237. www.cancer.gov.
- **National Coalition for Cancer Survivorship.** Furnishes publications, newsletter, education regarding the disease, insurance and legal rights. Networks, acts as advocate and clearinghouse. (877) 622-7937. www.canceradvocacy.org.
- **National Comprehensive Center Network (NCCN).** Alliance of 21 cancer centers offers guidelines to help patients and health professionals make informed decisions about cancer care. (215) 690-0300. www.nccn.com.
- **National Institutes of Health.** Medical research agency of the federal government delivers a cancer hotline. (800) 422-6237. www.nih.gov.
- **SHARE.** Hotline helps those affected by breast and ovarian cancers. (866) 891-2392. www.sharecancersupport.org.
- **Susan G. Komen For The Cure.** Has raised more than $1 billion for research, supports education, screening and treatment projects. Supplies hotline and 16-page booklet, "What's Happening to the Woman I Love? Couples Coping With Breast Cancer," a guide (in English or Spanish) for partners. (877) 465-6636. www.komen.org.

- "Uplift: Secrets from the Sisterhood of Breast Cancer," by Barbara Delinsky. Fifth anniversary edition, with new foreword. 336 pages. Paperback. $15. Washington Square Press, 2003. Practical (sometimes amusing) tips and anecdotes on daily life with the disease.
- **Women's Cancer Network.** Website developed by The Foundation for Women's Cancer, formerly the Gynecologic Center Foundation. Provides information, including links to news stories, via CancerSource, a clearinghouse. (800) 444-4441. www.wcn.org.
- **Young Survival Coalition.** Focuses on challenges faced by women 40 and under with breast cancer. (877) 972-1011. www.youngsurvival.org.

THE AUTHOR'S BIOGRAPHY

WOODY WEINGARTEN can't remember a time when he couldn't talk — or play with words.

His first poem was published in high school, but when his hormones announced that adulthood had arrived, he decided he'd rather eat than create rhymes (or even blank verse).

So he switched to journalism

And whadda ya know, the bearded, bespectacled guy has used big, small and hyphenated words professionally since jumpstarting his career in New Yawk City almost 60 years ago.

Today he's an author, columnist, reviewer-critic and blogger — despite allegedly being retired.

During his better-paid years as a wage slave, he was an executive editor and writer for daily and weekly publications in California, Florida, New Jersey, Pennsylvania and New York for more than five decades.

He won writing awards for public service and investigative pieces, features, columns, editorials and news.

In collaboration with his wife Nancy Fox, who's now been free of breast cancer for 20 years, he's completed an original musical revue, "Touching Up the Gray," which is still in need of a producer.

Woody, whose previous wife died when her breast cancer spread to vital organs, also has published weekly and monthly newspapers, and written a national column for "Audio" magazine.

A graduate of Colgate University, he owned a public relations/ad agency, directed a congressional primary campaign, served as media liaison for a psychiatric hospital, managed an advertising publication, and worked as a legislative aide.

The father of two and grandfather of three, he's lived in San Anselmo, California, for 28 years.

He figures he'll stay.

DEDICATION

This book is dedicated with tenderness and affection to:

- Nancy Fox, my soulmate, wife, friend and companion who supported this project even when it crossed the line of intimacy and took forever to finish.
- Irving N. Weingarten, my father-hero who up to his dying breath was convinced I should write a book — though I suspect he would have preferred a less weighty volume than this.
- Matilda Weingarten, my mother whose immense strength I failed to see until her final years.
- Janis L. Brown and Mark D. Weingarten, my daughter and son, who consistently gave me love and admiration, even when I occasionally handed them inflexibility.
- Zachary Weingarten and Drew Brown, my grandsons, and Hannah Schifrin, my granddaughter, who have brought me pleasure upon joy upon delight.
- Laura Schifrin, Hannah's mom, who generously sanctioned tons of time — which meant gobs of fun — for me to spend with her effervescent kid.
- Marv Edelstein, Dan Goltz, Heinz Feldman, John Teasley and the other Man to Man regulars and drop-ins who for decades endured my incessant chatter.
- Edward Marson, whose artistry is responsible for the graphic design of this book's covers; Larry Rosenberg, whose photo made me more pensive than ever; Alan Babbitt, whose back-cover shot lovingly captured Nancy and me lovingly staring at each other; and Wayne Heuring and Steve Cook for proofreading

and copy-editing "Rollercoaster" and making me re-look at every word, especially a few tortured metaphors and similes.

- Charlie Durden, a friend I will always miss, who vanished from my life one day into the L.A. smog — and died.
- All those buddies, acquaintances, relatives and colleagues I haven't cited by name who helped me and Nance through the breast-cancer years (as well as after and before).
- Each and every caregiver and patient forced to ride in a cancer rollercoaster.

Woody Weingarten
San Anselmo, California
Nov. 1, 2014

www.ingramcontent.com/pod-product-compliance
Lightning Source LLC
Chambersburg PA
CBHW032043040426
42334CB00038B/572